PEARLS FROM THE GOLDEN CABINET

PEARLS FROM

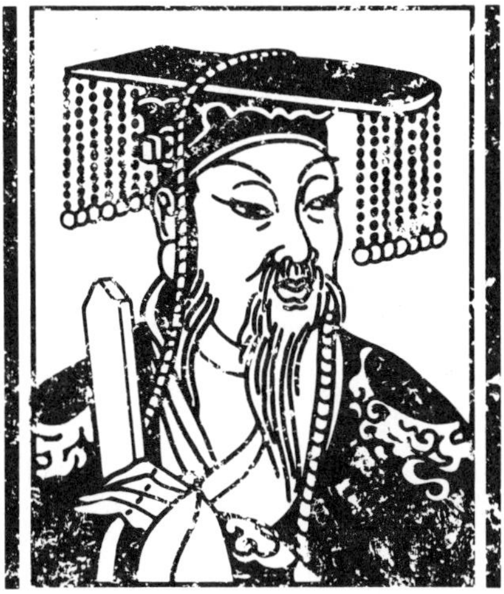

THE GOLDEN CABINET

The Practitioner's Guide To
The Use Of Chinese Herbs And
Traditional Formulas

by
Subhuti Dharmananda, Ph.D.

Library of Congress Catalog Card Number: 88-92366
ISBN: 0-941942-27-9

Manufactured in the United States of America

Published by Oriental Healing Arts Institute
1945 Palo Verde Avenue, Suite 208, Long Beach, CA 90815

Library of Congress Catalog in Publication Data
Dharmananda, Subhuti
Pearls from the Golden Cabinet
Bibliography: back cover
Includes indexes.
1. Herbs—Therapeutic use. 2. Materia medica—China. 3. Medicine, Chinese. I. Title.
(DNLM: 1. Drugs, Chinese Herbal. 2. Medicine, Chinese Traditional. WB 925 D533p)

RM666.H33D48 1988 615'.321'0951 88-92366
ISBN 0-941942-27-9

CONTENTS

INTRODUCTION 11

HARMONIZING FORMULAS
Bupleurum Formulas 33
Minor Bupleurum Combination 36
Bupleurum and Cinnamon Combination 38
Bupleurum and Cyperus Combination 40
Bupleurum, Cinnamon, and Ginger Combination 42
Bupleurum and Pinellia Combination 44
Bupleurum and Dragon Bone Combination 46
Major Bupleurum Combination 48
Bupleurum and Pueraria Combination 50
Bupleurum and Rehmannia Combination 52
Bupleurum and Chih-shih Combination 54
Bamboo and Ginseng Combination 56
Bupleurum and Peony Combination 58
Bupleurum Formula 60
Bupleurum and Magnolia Combinatin 61
Bupleurum and Ginseng Combination 62
Bupleurum and Evodia Combination 64

CHI TONIC AND DIGESTIVE FORMULAS
Ginseng Formulas 67
Four Major Herbs Combination 70
Six Major Herbs Combination 72
Ginseng and Tang-kuei Ten Combination 74
Pinellia Combination 76
Major Siler Combination 78
Ginseng Nutritive Combination 80
Ginseng and Longan Combination 82

Ginseng and Zizyphus Formula 84
Tang-kuei Sixteen Herb Combination 86

SURFACE RELIEVING AND RESPIRATIVE FORMULAS
Ma-Huang Formulas 89
Ma-huang, Licorice, and Apricot Seed Combination 91
Pueraria Combination 92
Minor Blue Dragon Combination 94
Ma-huang and Ginkgo Combination 96
Coix Combination 98
Cinnamon and Anemarrhena Combination 100

Purge Fire, Dispel Wind Formulas 103
Minor Rhubarb Combination 106
Gypsum Combination 108
Lonicera and Forsythia Combination 110
Pueraria Nasal Combination 112
Gambir Formula 114
Coptis and Scute Combination 116
Tang-kuei and Anemarrhena Combination 118
Astragalus and Atractylodes Combination 120
Gentiana Combination 122
Pueraria and Carthamus Combination 124
Ophiopogon and Asarum Combination 126
Tang-kuei and Arctium Combination 128
Siler and Platycodon Combination 130
Scute and Cimicifuga Combination 132
Gardenia and Vitex Combination 134
Lithospermum and Oyster Shell Combination 136
Magnolia and Gypsum Combination 138
Bupleurum and Schizonepeta Combination 139

Yin Tonic Formulas 141
Phellodendron Combination 144
Rehmannia Six Formula 146
Lycium Formula 148
Lily Combination 150
Platycodon and Fritillaria Combination 152
Tang-kuei and Rehmannia Combination 154
Cnidium and Moutan Combination 156
Ophiopogon Combination 158

Blood Activating Formulas 159
Moutan and Persica Combination 161

CONTENTS

Tang-kuei Four Combination 162
Cinnamon and Hoelen Formula 164
Clematis and Stephania Combination 166
Cinnamon and Persica Combination 168
Angelica and Mastic Combination 170
Cnidium and Rehmannia Combination 172

Moisture Moving Formulas 174
Vitality Combination 176
Hoelen Five Herb Formula 178
Stephania and Astragalus Combination 180
Polyporus Combination 181
Pinellia and Magnolia Combination 182
Pinellia and Gastrodia Combination 183
Citrus and Pinellia Combination 184

Herb Substitution Guide 187
Herb Name Index 190
Sympton Index 195
Formula Index 201
About Dosages 207

PREFACE

Herbal medicine has been practiced in the Orient for thousands of years. Sadly, though, it is barely known here in the West. Since former President Richard Nixon's visit to China in 1972, acupuncture has gained considerable acceptance in the United States, yet the Western medical and scientific community has never seriously considered the Oriental medical tradition and culture from which this discipline sprang.

About 1800 years ago, one of the greatest physicians in Chinese history, Zhang Zhong Jing, synthesized all the medical writings to date and incorporated his own empirical theories in the *Shang Han Za Bing Lun (Treatise on Febrile and Miscellaneous Diseases),* which was later divided into two important books, *Shang Han Lun* and *Jin Kui Yao Lue.* These two books have been translated to English recently and published by the Oriental Healing Arts Institute.

As these two classics show, Oriental medicine stresses reinforcing body resistance to eliminate pathogens. It is a preventive medicine in which diseases are diagnosed and treated at the early indications so that they can be deterred from entering the later stages. Although modern Western medicine has made great contributions to the treatment of many diseases, its therapeutic methods often produce side effects. Some authorities estimate that Western drugs cause side effects in 20 percent of all cases. This problem is further compounded by the burgeoning cost of modern medical care. If present trends continue, by 1990, 20 percent of America's gross national product will go towards medical bills.

To help lessen side effects and reduce costs, we have dedicated ourselves to introducing Oriental Medicine to the

United States. In August of 1980, I visited the author in Santa Cruz, California and was pleased to find him knowledgeable in both science and Oriental Medicine. Since then our friendship has grown, in part through our mutual recognition of the importance of Chinese medicine to the well-being of Western society.

Dr. Dharmananda has travelled extensively in the Orient. He has visited the Brion Research Institute and the Sun Ten Pharmaceutical Company in Taipei, Taiwan, where he observed firsthand scientific herbal research and processing methods. He has spoken at the Chinese University in Hong Kong and visited the People's Republic of China a number of times.

The author has selected 70 herbal formulas especially suitable for treating the more common ailments of Western society. He and his colleagues have demonstrated the effectiveness of these formulas through clinical experiences. His book tells the reader why, how, and when to use Chinese herbal formulas, as well as how formulas can be modified to suit a patient's particular conformation. It includes a section defining some of the more important Chinese medical terms, and also explains some of the more significant pulse and tongue symptoms.

Pearls from the Golden Cabinet is concise and practical, an indispensable guide for professional and non-professional herbalists who wish to prescribe herbal formulas effectively. Undoubtedly, this book will promote holistic healing and further the understanding of traditional Chinese medicine, which views the human body and disease from a viewpoint very different from that of Western medicine. I hope that traditional Chinese medicine will not only provide an alternative way to fight diseases and promote health, but also reduce the soaring cost of health care in the West.

Hong-yen Hsu, Ph.D.
President,
Oriental Healing Arts Institute
January 1988

INTRODUCTION

Chinese herbalists frequently produce an herbal prescription that is carefully tailored to the needs of the patient at the time. Extensive experience has shown, however, that certain patterns of disharmony appear over and over again among many different individuals and that certain combinations of herbs are particularly effective for treating each of those patterns. As a result, despite the ability of the herbalist to combine virtually any of several hundred herbs to produce a therapeutic formula, certain combinations of a more limited number of herbs appear repeatedly. In fact, the prescriptions are often drawn from a basic set of standard formulas which are modified only slightly, if at all, for the individual case at hand. A survey of practitioners reveals that about fifty to one hundred base formulas are adequate for the majority of applications. This book presents one selection of basic formulas and some of the ways in which they are likely to be modified.

Traditionally, most of the formulas described in this book were given as decoctions. Practitioners in the West often find that there is a significant problem with compliance when administering herbal decoctions—many of their clients dislike making and drinking the herb teas. The same problem exists in Asia, but to a lesser extent simply because the tradition of taking strong teas is so prevalent. Herbalists attempt to minimize the use of decoctions by offering powders or pills for long term administration following a period of a few days' or weeks' use of the teas.

Fortunately, these traditional Chinese formulas are now readily available in the form of scientifically prepared concentrated extracts which have proven popular in Asia and the West. The efficacy, versatility in making prescriptions, and price of the concentrated extracts is comparable with that of crude herbs used to make decoctions. This book can be used in working with either these modern extract granules or the more traditional decoctions and powders made from crude herbs.

ABOUT THE TITLE

In 206 B.C., Liu Pang founded the great Han Dynasty. The Chinese people so loved this compassionate leader that all future generations of Chinese have called themselves the sons of Han. It was during the 430 years of the Han Dynasty that the diverse knowledge of Chinese herbal medicine, gathered since time immemorial, was consolidated and formalized. *The Herbal of Shen Nong,* considered the first official pharmacopeia of China, was compiled around 100 A.D.; it included 365 famous Chinese herbs with descriptions of their features, growing location, time of harvest, and medicinal uses.

The renowned physician Zhang Zhong Jing wrote China's first herbal formulary at the close of the Han Dynasty period (220 A.D.). The original work was later divided into two books, the first known as the *Shang Han Lun (Discussion of Febrile Diseases),* and the second known as *Jin Kui Yao Lue (Prescriptions from the Golden Cabinet).* These works remain among the most important medical texts of Chinese history and are still studied by medical students in the Orient.

The Golden Cabinet represents a repository of precious prescriptions. Zhang contributed more than 250 formulas to initiate the collection. Hundreds of other efficacious prescriptions have been added by physicians working in China and Japan during the past seventeen centuries. All these formulas have been well-tested and proven by the experiences of millions of people.

Pearls symbolize precious things that are compact, simple, and smooth; their value increases with time, and their appearance is formal and glowing. The formulas described in this guide are simple, yet sophisticated, remarkably effective, relatively easy to master, and they retain their usefulness over the centuries despite the changing nature of our environment and our diseases. They serve to illuminate the methods of herbal prescribing and provide an understanding of other important traditional prescriptions.

HERBAL CONCENTRATES

A solution to the compliance problems often associated with traditional herbal decoctions was achieved in Taiwan 40 years ago by the Sun Ten Pharmaceutical Works Co. Combining traditional herb knowledge, modern technologies, and the results of pharmacologic research, Sun Ten now turns Chinese herbal decoctions into a concentrated extract powder or granule that can be taken easily.

The herbs (stored in refrigerated warehouses) are cooked according to ancient methods in giant vats. The resulting tea is gently heated in a chamber and the essential oils are collected. The remaining tea is carefully cooked down to produce a syrup, which is then spray-dried to make granules. The essential oils are added back. The use of sealed chambers, low pressure, low temperatures, the separation of the essential oil fraction, and stringent quality control measures assure that virtually nothing is lost. The resulting product is quite similar in content, but not form, to the decoction made at home, and may be superior because patients may not be as careful in preparing the decoction as the practitioner would like.

Sun Ten's research arm, the Brion Research Institute, was established in 1972 by Dr. Hong-yen Hsu, and currently employs 50 researchers. The Institute has a large library, a repository of some 3000 herb samples and 5000 herbarium specimens, a comprehensive chemistry laboratory, several analytical laboratories, and an animal research area for pharmacological testing. It is the largest medicinal plants research institute in Taiwan.

The researchers are involved in a wide range of studies. A primary research objective is to identify the most suitable herbal materials for use in traditional Chinese herb formulas manufactured by Sun Ten Pharmaceutical Works. Important to this process is the identification of the original plant materials found in the Chinese markets using histologic, morphologic, and other botanical means; to isolate, identify, and quantify the major active constituents; and to test the plant materials and their constituents for pharmacological activity in animal studies (usually using mice and rabbits). Thus, an investigation might begin with identifying a dozen herbs sold on the market under the same traditional name (and thus interchanged by herbalists who apply them for the same use), and end with the knowledge that one of these herb samples, processed by specific methods, produces the most sought-after effects.

Brion Research Institute collects data which is presented to the authorities in Taiwan and in Japan in order to license the Sun Ten Pharmaceutical products for sale in those countries. About four years of work is required to obtain a license for one of the formulas. The concentrated extracts made by Sun Ten include more than 375 individual herbs and about 337 traditional Chinese herbal formulas. The Ministry of Health and Welfare of the Japanese government has established guidelines for approving Chinese herb formulas; the approved formulas are covered by national health insurance. Thus far, more than 148 of the traditional Chinese herb formulas have been approved. Further, the Japanese Pharmaceutical Manufacturers Joint Committee on Medicine has evaluated the question of quality control and established guidelines. When a manufacturer outside of Japan wishes to submit a product for import, it must first undergo extensive testing and the results are evaluated by a Japanese government committee. Thus far, eighty of the Sun Ten formulas have been evaluated and accepted by Japan. According to their rating system, Sun Ten products rank among the highest quality compared to those of the twenty major manufacturers in Japan.

The degree of concentration of the granules is standardized so that the daily dosage for each formula is about the same: 4.5-6.0 grams per day (a level teaspoon is about 3 grams). This represents approximately one-half the dosage administered to patients in a Chinese hospital or clinic. If desired, one can take up to three times as much for a short period of treatment, such as during acute stages of an illness. For long-term administration and for individuals who are more sensitive to the effects of herbs, a dosage of 2.0-4.0 grams of concentrate per day is adequate and cost-effective.

METHODS OF ADMINISTRATION

The decoctions, when made from good quality materials and properly cooked to preserve the active constituents, are considered by many practitioners to be the most efficacious way to give herbs;

but they are only useful when the person takes them as directed. The reason for the rapid and strong response to the teas is not so much that they are prepared in the liquid form as that it is common for the dosage of herbs used in making the teas to be relatively high. In fact, it is standard procedure to use up to three times the dosage of crude herbs in making a medicinal tea compared to other forms of the herbs.

The prepared concentrated extracts, made from very high-quality materials and processed with care, are similarly efficacious and more likely to be taken as directed. The dosage of crude herbs used for making the daily dose of extracts is comparable to that used in making a moderate dosage herb tea, but may be less than that prescribed in Oriental hospitals.

An objection to any prepared formula is that it cannot be altered to suit the individual. However, because extracts of single herbs are also available in the form of concentrates, they can be added to the base formula to make a new, personalized prescription.

The patent formula pills that are often available from Chinese herb shops are sometimes also made from concentrated extracts, but they are not as suitable for clinical use because the formula cannot be altered. They are often inexpensive, easy to administer, and thus suitable for long-term use or for a brief trial period of a particular therapeutic approach.

HOW TO USE THIS BOOK

The purpose of this book is to aid the practitioner in selecting the most suitable formula using the standard diagnostic features of Traditional Chinese Medicine rather than Western style indications. Since it is usual practice to adjust a formula to the needs of the individual, examples of typical variations from the standard formulas are described. When using the extract granules, about 10-15 grams of each single herb granule is added to a packet of 100 grams of the base formula. In that way, the added herb comprises approximately 8-10% of the finished formula. This is an average amount, since most traditional prescriptions contain about ten to twelve ingredients.

Each page of the formula section is devoted to one primary

formula, but a number of other formulas are mentioned in the text (their names in bold print). In the majority of cases, the other formulas are made from the primary formula by adding a few single herbs; the resulting formula may be described in detail as a primary formula on another page. The formula names that head each page, as well as others mentioned in the text, are those used by the Oriental Healing Arts Institute in their books *Commonly Used Chinese Herb Formulas with Illustrations* and *Natural Healing with Chinese Herbs.* Just below the heading, the Pinyin transliteration of the Chinese name is provided. When the original Chinese name for the formula has a meaning describing its use, the literal translation is also given. Dr. Hsu has translated the Chinese word "tang" (literal: soup or decoction) as "combination", and has used the word "formula" for all other designations such as "san" (powder), "wan" (pill), "yin" (special medicine), or "dan" (elixir). Generally, the English formula name developed by Dr. Hsu is based on the "Emperor" of the formula—that is, the herb or pair of herbs that determines the primary therapeutic functions of the formula. These formula names are used throughout the publications of the Oriental Healing Arts Institute and the Institute for Traditional Medicine.

PATHOLOGY TERMINOLOGY

The action of each formula is presented briefly in a section on therapeutic principles in terms of Traditional Chinese Medicine. Because each traditionally defined action has many physiologic implications, it is easy to give a short description for a formula that has many diverse uses.

Unfortunately, the terminology used by Chinese doctors has not been translated in a consistent manner. For the sake of consistency within this book, an explanation of terms which are similar but which have important, subtle differences is provided in the following section on Terminology. These definitions do not necessarily follow those used by other authors, but they have been made as close as possible to the definitions appearing in frequently used texts.

INTRODUCTION; PATHOLOGY TERMINOLOGY

I. Distinguishing Dampness and Moisture:

DAMPNESS is localized fluid accumulation associated with pathology of the tissues. It is often associated with heat (damp-heat) or disturbed organ function (e.g. damp Spleen syndrome).

MOISTURE is one of the three humors of Chinese medical doctrine. Accumulation of Moisture produces general swelling. It is often associated with cold syndromes, and deficient function (Yang) of the Spleen and Kidney. Excessive Moisture is often discharged via frequent urination and loose stool.

Dampness and Moisture accumulation may occur simultaneously. Abdominal bloating, or muscular and articular swelling and numbness are usually treated by moving Moisture; leukorrhea or skin eruptions with pus are treated by drying dampness or "purging damp-heat." Both conditions may be treated with herbs that benefit the condition of the Spleen and Kidney, two organs especially important in removing Moisture.

II. Distinguishing Wind and Internal Wind:

WIND refers to external factors that cause surface pain (e.g. headache and arthralgia), surface fever (e.g. colds, flus, and skin eruptions), or surface congestion (e.g. muscular tension and general aching). It may be associated with heat (wind-heat) or cold (wind-chill).

INTERNAL WIND refers to a Liver disorder which produces nervous problems such as twitching, convulsions, vertigo, muscular tension, ringing in the ears, paralysis, etc. Internal wind, sometimes called "draft," is often associated with fire. The syndrome may be related to excess Chi of the Liver or deficiency of Blood and/or Yin reducing the ability of the Liver to regulate the Chi.

Internal wind and 'external' wind may occur simultaneously, as with headaches focused over the eyes, shoulder/neck tension, skin itching, and contractile pain in the limbs. Invasion of wind and congestion of the surface is treated with diaphoretic formulas that dispel wind, while internal wind is treated with Liver-relieving and sedative formulas that often contain fire-purging herbs. Herbs for treating rheumatism and skin-itching are often useful in treating both internal and external wind factors.

III. Distinguishing Stagnant Blood and Blood Stasis:

STAGNANT BLOOD is Blood that is flowing weakly through an area, providing it with less than adequate nutrition. Blood stagnation is most common in the lower abdomen and is often associated with the menstrual system. Blood stagnation is usually related to deficiency of Chi and cold blockage.

BLOOD STASIS refers to Blood that is clotted in the capillary beds (it may also clot in the arteries). Blood stasis leads to localized heat syndromes and the production of tumors, cysts, boils, and other swellings. It is evidenced by sharp pain and the appearance of purple color in the tongue. It may also have systemic effects with symptoms related to Blood heat, such as skin eruptions and headaches. New Blood cannot be properly formed when there is stasis. The term "ecchymosis entity" has been applied to clotted Blood. Stasis usually occurs in areas of circulatory complexity, such as the joints, the female reproductive organs, the breast, the brain, and the heart.

Blood stagnancy and Blood stasis may occur simultaneously, but the symptoms of Blood stasis (e.g. heat syndrome and sharp pain) will predominate in such circumstances. Menstrual irregularity and chronic vaginal infection are often attributed to stagnant Blood and are treated by mild herbs that promote blood circulation. Severe menstrual pain, severe joint pains, and tumors are often attributed to Blood stasis and are treated by strong herbs that dispel Blood stasis and activate Blood circulation (sometimes called "ABC agents").

IV. Distinguishing Phlegm and Sputum:

PHLEGM is used here as the most general term; phlegm can refer to sputum or it can refer to substances that affect the mind, nerves, lymph system, skin, and joints. The latter is usually associated with a fire syndrome, often deficiency fire; phlegm is a heat-congealed fluid. Phlegm is treated by aromatics (such as borneol), certain animal parts (e.g. silkworm and gallstones), and some minerals, as well as by standard herbal phlegm resolvers (e.g. pinellia, laminaria, and fritillaria).

SPUTUM refers to the abnormal secretions of the lungs. Sputum is treated by herbs that dissolve phlegm (usually acrid herbs), relieve the coughing reflex (anti-tussive action), and by expectorants (herbs that aid the movement of sputum). Excessive sputum is dried up by astringent herbs.

Sputum and other types of phlegm congestion may occur simultaneously. These conditions tend to be marked by a greasy tongue coating and a pearl-like or congested pulse. Disorders of the lungs, sinuses, ears, and lymph glands are often treated with warm, acrid herbs that dispel wind, move Moisture, and dissolve phlegm (they may be matched with cold bitter herbs and cold acrid herbs for treating heat syndromes). Coughing and wheezing is treated with anti-tussives and expectorants. Disorders of the mind, nerves, and joints (these are usually severe disorders with degeneration of tissues) are usually treated by aromatics and animal drugs that resolve heated phlegm. Phlegm and sputum syndromes are often treated by warming the Gallbladder (improving digestion of fats and dispersing stagnant energy).

V. Distinguishing Fire, Heat, and Toxins:

FIRE refers to an internal condition related to excess Yang or deficient Yin of one or more organ systems; the result is excessive or uncontrolled Chi. Fire usually produces redness, pressure, and excitability. By convention, fire syndromes are associated with the Liver, Heart, Kidney, and Stomach.

HEAT refers to a condition of the Blood or the body's surface. Heat of the Blood produces a tendency towards itching, burning, or inflamed skin or mucus membranes (in the latter case, usually called "damp-heat"). By convention, heat syndromes are associated with the Gallbladder, Bladder, and Spleen (all as damp-heat) and with the Lung.

TOXINS may occur in the Blood (one component of "Blood

heat") or associated with an inflammatory process (infection).

Fire, heat, and toxins may occur simultaneously; for example, sore throat and acne represent heat in the Upper Warmer and often arise when the person has Liver and Heart fire; there are toxins produced by the infecting organisms, and there may be toxins in the Blood that were partly responsible for initiating the infection. Fire is purged by cold, bitter herbs; heat is relieved by cool, acrid herbs or by herbs that act on the Blood; toxins are cleared or the Blood is detoxified.

VI. Distinguishing Deficiency States:

WEAKNESS of an organ system refers to any deficiency state associated with it. The weak system is not capable of responding correctly to various stressful stimuli.

DEFICIENCY OF YANG OR CHI refers to the condition in which the body is unable to provide adequate warmth, metabolic function, and movement of Chi, Moisture, and Blood.

DEFICIENCY OF YIN, BLOOD, OR ESSENCE occurs when any of these basic substances are lacking.

These different types of deficiency syndromes often occur together. The predominant type(s) of deficiency will determine the main therapeutic techniques to be employed. Organ systems are strengthened, Yang and Chi are tonified, Yin and Blood are nourished. Generally, whenever Yin, Blood, or Essence is nourished, it is also important to tonify Chi and Yang, and vice versa.

INDICATIONS FOR USE

The Chinese system of diagnosis relies primarily upon questioning (which provides a list of subjective symptoms), pulse diagnosis, and examination of the tongue. The descriptions under the heading "Indications for Use" include a list of typical symptoms and occasionally Western disease names. Throughout this book, traditional Chinese medical terms for organs and primary humors have a capital letter. For more information about Chinese diagnostic terminology, please consult THE WEB THAT HAS NO WEAVER by Ted Kaptchuk, O.M.D., and publications by the Oriental Healing Arts Institute.

The indications for use are not intended to be comprehensive, as the Chinese herb formulas can be applied to all cases calling for the therapeutic principles involved. Instead, the indications listed in this book are examples of conditions for which the formula is considered suitable when the individual taking the herb formula has the correct qualifications (called "conformation").

PULSE CATEGORIES

While it is relatively easy to describe the meaning of a particular pulse, it is quite difficult to say what kinds of pulses are likely to indicate the use of a particular formula. This is because the pulse is just one of many pieces of information and there are many complicating factors that would produce different pulses. By using very broad pulse categories to aid in matching this diagnostic feature with formula indications, one can suggest the pulse type that is likely. It is usually not possible to be more specific. Even these broad categories must be regarded as only suggestive.

FLOATING: felt easily at the surface—usually indicates some surface involvement in the disease process; typical in early stage of colds and flus (invasion of wind) and with excess type disorders; it may also occur when there is a collapse of Yang. This pulse type is sometimes called "superficial."

SINKING: felt with deep palpation—usually indicates that the body's energy is constrained to the interior; typical when there is constipation, Blood stasis, or significant weakness of one or more organ systems.

THIN: the width of the pulse under the finger is less than average —usually indicates that there is a deficiency of Yin; common with thirst, dry skin, constipation, etc. When the pulse is also weak, it is sometimes designated as "thready."

FULL: the width of the pulse under the fingers is greater than average, and the pulse retains strength and form when more pressure is applied—usually indicates an excess condition requiring purgation or dispersing therapies.

TENSE: feels like a bowstring and presents some force—usually indicates Liver tension; it is common with restrained anger. This pulse is sometimes designated as "wiry."

FAST: the pulse rate is greater than about 4-5 beats per respiration —usually indicates a heat syndrome; there are often inflammatory processes underway. A strong or full pulse that is fast indicates heat thriving; a thin or weak pulse that is fast suggests Yin deficiency.

SLOW: the pulse rate is 4 or fewer beats per respiration—usually indicates a cold syndrome or strong stagnancy of circulation; there may be pain, lethargy, or chill.

SLIPPERY: the pulse is firm and round, feeling like pearls under the fingers—usually indicates phlegm accumulation, but may also occur with stagnation of Moisture; the tongue coating, if present, is usually greasy; the lungs and sinuses may be congested; the digestion disturbed; in severe cases, the nerves may show damage or the mind may be disturbed. A slippery pulse is normal during the second to eighth week of pregnancy.

CONGESTED: this is a term used in this book to account for several traditional categories; the pulse has a slippery quality, but it is sinking and may not fill the three-finger pulse taking segment (the "Kidney pulses" are either weak or absent)—usually indicates congestion of Phlegm or Blood with deficiency of Yin; there may be a variety of abdominal disturbances.

SOFT: the pulse spreads and moves with pressure—usually indicates accumulation of Moisture; the Spleen and Kidney may be weak.

WEAK: the pulse is difficult to detect, it may be thready, or it disappears with pressure—usually indicates a Weak Constitution or a deficiency of Chi and Blood; there may also be deficiencies of Yang and Yin. The voice is usually weak, and the individual may appear pale and deficient.

STRONG: the pulse has good form and resilience, indicating a Strong Constitution and no major deficiency; it is typical of a healthy individual or one who usually recovers easily from illness.

TONGUE DESIGNATIONS

The tongue is said to be the "sprout of the Heart" and it reveals the condition of the Blood. The designations include:

PALE: weak circulation (deficiency of Yang or Chi, weakness of Heart, or constrained (Chi and Blood), deficiency of Blood (anemia and other deficiency states).

RED: Blood heat, deficiency of Yin, fire of Heart or Liver, toxic blood states.

PURPLE SPOTS: Blood stasis (usually shows up as small areas of purplish hue).

The coating of the tongue is said to be from "mist of the Spleen" and it reveals the condition of the digestive system. The designations include:

WHITE COATING: this is normal; it becomes more pronounced when there is coldness or obstruction of energy flow, and it also thickens in the early phase of a surface disorder (such as cold or flu).

YELLOW COATING: this indicates heat originating from or entering the digestive system; frequently accompanies constipation, Liver fire, chronic infections, etc.

NO COATING: occurs when the Spleen is very weak (in which case, the tongue is usually moist), and when there is severe deficiency of Yin (the tongue is dry).

Other factors important in tongue diagnosis include the texture and moistness of the tongue and coating:

DRY TONGUE: indicates Yin deficiency or imbalance of water metabolism.

MOIST TONGUE: indicates Spleen dampness or deficiency of Yang.

GREASY COATING OR CREAMY COATING: indicates phlegm accumulation.

SWOLLEN TONGUE: when pale, usually indicates accumulation of Moisture; when red, indicates excess heat condition.

SHRUNKEN TONGUE: indicates deficiency of Yin and Blood; occurs after a prolonged fire syndrome.

TONGUE WON'T PROTRUDE: usually indicates Liver tension.

TONGUE QUIVERS: usually indicates internal wind or weak Spleen Chi or both.

CRACKS IN TONGUE: usually indicates long-term deficiency syndrome.

RED DOTS AT TIP: suggests excess Heart fire (if they are prominent).

RED DOTS EXTENDING TO SIDE: suggests Liver fire.

RAISED BUMPS AT BACK OF TONGUE: usually indicates Kidney fire.

For a detailed description of tongue diagnosis, see TONGUE DIAGNOSIS IN CHINESE MEDICINE by Giovanni Maciocia and a book on the same subject by Dr. Ze-lin Chen and Dr. Mei-fang Chen (publication in progress for a 1988 release by the Oriental Healing Arts Institute).

THE ROLE OF INDIVIDUAL HERBS IN A FORMULA

Below each formula description is a direct presentation of

the formula ingredients, using English and Pinyin names, with dosage indicated in grams per day (use Chien per day for making decoctions; 1 Chien equals about three grams). This information is taken directly from *Commonly Used Herb Formulas with Illustrations and Natural Healing with Chinese Herbs.*

The herbs are divided into subgroups according to therapeutic role and major organ system affected. The complete lists of herbal ingredients are mentioned also in the section on Herbs and Actions. Of course, each herb often has several roles; an interpretation of the main role is given. In some cases, two different aspects of the herb's action is suggested in relation to its interactions with other herbs in the formula. The division of herbs into groups differs between the Herbs and Actions section and the listing of ingredients given below it so as to provide two different perspectives by which to understand the formula.

The English names of herbs used throughout this text are the same as those used by the Oriental Healing Arts Institute, which were developed by the following basic rules:

1) If a common name has long been in existence, it is retained; e.g. licorice, jujube, and ginger.

2) If no English common name has been available or the name is rarely used, the genus name of the plant becomes the common name; e.g. bupleurum, coptis, and pinellia.

3) If several species of the same genus are commonly used in Chinese medicine, one plant may receive the genus name while all others are designated by their transliterated Chinese name (simplified Wade-Giles system). For example, angelica, tang-kuei, and tu-huo are designations for three different species of angelica.

In the back of this book, there is a cross-reference table of these common names, the Pinyin, and the pharmaceutical names. The advantage of using the English names is that it becomes relatively easy for English-speaking people to discuss the herbs; the pharmaceutical names are often too clumsy and the Pinyin is difficult to pronounce properly unless one has mastered the Chinese language.

ALTERING THE BASE FORMULAS

In the section on Typical Variations, examples of herbs that can be added to the base formula to emphasize specific actions, or to add new actions, are given. Whenever possible, traditional formulas (which are named in bold type) are mentioned if they can be produced from the formula under discussion by relatively simple modification. Most of these formulas are also available in the form of concentrated extract granules, usually with all the herbs cooked together (sometimes the supplier must modify a base formula when the desired item is not in stock). One aim of this book is to permit the construction of numerous traditional formulas using extract granules without requiring the practitioner to stock all of them. A collection of single herb granules (which are always desirable for formula personalization) and a relatively small number of base formulas is usually adequate.

In the event that a desired single herb granule is not on hand, a substitute might be used. In the Appendix, a list of typical substitutions is presented.

FORMULA SIZE

Formulas developed during the Han, Tang, and Sung Dynasties and the brief Dynastic periods in between (206 B.C. to 1279 A.D.) were usually comprised of a relatively small number of herbs (typically 4-9 herbs) which were arranged in a large variety of ways. For example, in the *Shang Han Lun* and *Jin Kui Yao Lue* (ca. 220 A.D.), there are more than a dozen chill-dispelling formulas with just 4-6 herbs in each that are comprised of various combinations of ginseng, cinnamon, aconite, ginger, atractylodes, hoelen, peony, jujube, and licorice.

It is possible to combine two or more of these short formulas, or to add two to four herbs to these formulas in order to make treatments specific for an individual or a particular type of ailment. It is easy to add entirely new, but related, therapeutic principles to the action of the original formula. For example, one may combine the Spleen strengthening formula FourMajor Herbs Combination with the Blood nourishing formula Tang-kuei Four Combination to produce the nutritive Tang-kuei and Ginseng Eight Combination. Alternatively, one may combine the fire-purging Coptis and Scute Combination with Tang-kuei Four Combination in order to produce Tang-kuei and Gardenia Combination which then cools the Blood and treats uterine bleeding and skin disorders. A characteristic of most of these early formulas is that they are very malleable to adjustment.

In later Dynasties, such as the Yuan, Ming, and Qing (1260-1911 A.D.) much larger formulas became popular. These typically had 10-18 herbs each, and in some cases they were made by combining portions of two or three ancient formulas and then making a few modifications. These formulas are quite specific and, generally speaking, one does not modify them except to add one or two herbs to emphasize one of the therapeutic principles already contained in the formula. It is usually much more difficult to redirect the actions of these larger formulas.

CHOICE OF FORMULAS AND DIVISION INTO CATEGORIES

Seventy basic formulas that are most representative of the available combinations were selected for inclusion in this work. Through discussion of other traditional formulas produced by making various additions, the total number of formulas described comes to more than one hundred and forty. Acupuncturists, herbalists, and other health practitioners can satisfy most needs of their clients using these formulas and their modifications. Of course, there are other formulas that might prove more suitable for particular patients, and the reader is directed to the resources mentioned in the bibliography for information about the other formulas. The formulas are divided into seven categories:

1) **HARMONIZING FORMULAS:** generally used for treating Liver-related disorders, digestive disturbances, and Lung diseases.

2) **CHI TONIC & DIGESTIVE FORMULAS:** generally for strengthening the Spleen, tonifying Chi, and nourishing Blood.

3) **BLOOD-CIRCULATING FORMULAS:** for treating Blood stasis, for nourishing Blood, and treating gynecologic problems.

4) **YIN TONIC FORMULAS:** to nourish the Yin and Blood, and relieve deficiency fire.

5) **FIRE PURGING AND WIND DISPELLING FORMULAS:** generally used for skin ailments, hypertension, obesity, constipation, inflammatory ailments, etc., but not for deficiency fire syndromes.

6) **SURFACE-RELIEVING & LUNG OPENING FORMULAS:** for treating asthma, cough, arthritis, and edema.

7) **MOISTURE MOVING FORMULAS:** used for edema, kidney and bladder disorders, and cold syndromes.

Many times, a formula in one category will also treat a variety of conditions that belong to other categories. For example, Bamboo and Ginseng Combinations is a harmonizing formula, a chi tonifying formula, and a fire purging formula.

Certain categories of formulas that might otherwise be logically included in such a list have been placed within the categories mentioned above. For example, Tang-kuei formulas are common, but most of them fit very easily into the harmonizing, chi tonifying, and blood circulating sections. Treatments for acute diseases fit mostly in the fire purging section. Yang tonics are not common in the form of extract formulas: there are several Yang tonic herbs in the Yin tonic section since these formulas are basic supplements to the Kidney. Thus, of the many possible therapeutic divisions, most are covered in the above seven sections.

SAFETY OF CHINESE HERBS

Chinese herb formulas are non-toxic and can be taken in quite large doses without toxic effects. Some Chinese herbs have been processed to eliminate most of their natural toxic component, as in the case of aconite and pinellia. One should be careful when using the single-herb granules of these slightly toxic herbs since it is possible to obtain a large dose of them by using the concentrated extracts. Some formulas may produce discomforts in certain individuals and the means of avoiding this are suggested in the introduction to each of the formula sections.

THE SERVANT HERBS

The actions of most Chinese formulas can be explained by describing the contributions of ingredients according to four categories: the EMPEROR (the herb or herbs that define the primary therapeutic principles), the MINISTERS (herbs that support and broaden the desired functions of the Emperor herb and counter effects that are not desired), the ASSISTANTS (herbs that make the formula more suitable for the constitution of the individual), and the SERVANTS. The functions of the servant herbs are to harmonize or coordinate the actions of the other herbs in the formula, direct the other herbs to act on a specific part of the body, improve the formula's overall effects, and sometimes to boost the Chi. In addition, they reduce the toxicity or harshness of the stronger herbs that are often used as Emperors and Ministers. The majority of traditional Chinese herb formulas utilize one or more servant herbs. The most common servant is licorice, which harmonizes the actions of the other herbs. The next most common is a combination of ginger, jujube, and licorice, which strengthens and normalizes the Stomach/Spleen, tonifies Chi, and aids in the treatment of acute ailments. Reference here to "acute ailments" is in contrast to "chronic ailments" and means a short-term ailment, such as cold, flu, headache , muscle spasm, or flare-up of symptoms associated with a chronic ailment.

In this book, the servant herbs are usually not assigned according to an organ system effect, though most act on the Spleen and Stomach.

RESPONSES TO THE USE OF HERBS

There are three types of responses usually encountered by persons using Chinese herb formulas:

1) The person feels much better taking the herbs, and the therapy is regarded as successful. In that case, the same formula or a very similar one should be taken until no further progress is made. Then, usually after a short period without using herbs, another evaluation should be made and a different formula given. This procedure is followed until it is decided that herbal therapies are no longer needed on a regular basis. As a rule, an individual should not take one herb formula consistently for more than a month without re-evaluation. The possible exception is long-term use of certain Kidney and Spleen tonics for chronic deficiency states.

2) The person claims that the herbs do nothing. One must check carefully for changes in symptomology to be sure that no changes have occurred, as reported. Some clients only look at one symptom to evaluate their progress even though other aspects of their disorder may be clearing up (e.g. a skin problem may not have changed, but the person is sleeping better, digesting foods better, and has more energy; perhaps it will take longer to see improvement in the skin). If, in fact, no changes have occurred, try the following procedures:

a) Re-evaluate the person's condition and consider whether or not the therapy is truly appropriate. Change the formula if necessary.

b) If the formula seems appropriate, re-evaluate the dosage and increase it. The Japanese dosage system (which is for gentle effects over a period of time) utilized in this text recommends about one-third the dosage used in China to produce more powerful effects over a shorter term of therapy.

c) If increasing the dosage does not produce an effect, consider using herbs of the same therapeutic principle that have a stronger action. Thus, hot, acrid, and very aromatic herbs usually have a stronger dispensing effect than warm, sweet, tonic herbs even though both may be indicated for aiding circulation of Chi and Moisture.

3) The person complains of adverse effects. If there are gastrointestinal disturbances, the herbs should be taken about an hour after meals rather than on an empty stomach; one may also add to the formula herbs that aid digestion and treat either diarrhea or constipation if either condition seems to develop as a result of herb use. In other cases of adverse reaction, it is possible that a therapy which is acting to disperse Chi, Moisture, or Blood encounters a weakness in some area of the body, and there is an intolerance to the stimulation. In such cases, the addition of tonic herbs and the reduction of dispersive, stimulating, and eliminative herbs should resolve the problem. Generally speaking, persons indicating adverse responses other than digestive disturbance require tonics for the Yin and/or Blood, and may also require sedatives for the Heart.

STORAGE OF CONCENTRATED EXTRACTS

Extract granules are usually supplied in 100 gram packets that can be most easily stored in file cabinets made for 4x6 cards. A heavy cardboard version of these cabinets is the least expensive, and a suitable method. If the formulas are stored alphabetically (or numerically), it is easy to find the desired one. The single herb granules should be transferred to bottles, since they will be used in small amounts frequently. A 300 cc. brown glass bottle will hold

100-150 grams of granules, depending upon the herb. When providing a modified formula to clients, the contents of the base formula packet can be poured into a sufficiently large empty bottle, the single-herb granules added, and after securing a lid on the bottle, it is shaken for a few seconds to mix all the granules. The resulting formula can be offered either in bottles or in plastic zip lock bags; it is best to double-bag in order to minimize the chance of loss due to puncture. For smaller amounts of herbs to be used for an acute condition, enough granules for two to three days use can be provided in 50 cc. bottles.

INTRODUCTION TO BUPLEURUM

Bupleurum was a favorite herb of Zhang Zhong Jing and many of his followers throughout the history of Traditional Chinese Medicine. Today it is the most popular herb in the Japanese Kanpo, and it is rapidly gaining acceptance in the West. Bupleurum is the primary herb of harmonization therapy, and is the most commonly used herb for treating Liver disorders classified under the headings constrained Liver Chi (Liver tension), internal wind, and Liver fire. For simplicity, in the description of therapeutic principles, the combined action of bupleurum on tension, internal wind, and fire are grouped under the heading **"relieve the Liver."**

The following are characteristic symptoms of constrained Liver Chi:

cold hands/feet
menstrual irregularity and pain
shoulder/neck tension, low back ache
nervousness, irritability
hypoglycemia and food allergy
depression
breast lumps and uterine tumors
ulcer and digestive disturbance
tendency to constipation
premenstrual tension
fatigue
tense pulse

If instead of constrained Liver Chi, the condition of Liver fire predominates, then the following kinds of symptoms arise:

hypertension
constipation
sinusitis
red eyes
bronchitis
skin eruption

headaches
facial flushing
hepatitis
excessive sweating
ringing in the ears
ulcer
insomnia
full pulse

The section on fire purging formulas should be consulted if these symptoms are predominant.

Internal wind is usually an accompanying condition rather than a primary one, giving rise to muscle tension and spasms, itching skin, migrating pains, and joint problems.

STANDARD MATCHING IN BUPLEURUM COMBINATIONS

In treating Liver problems, bupleurum is typically matched with other herbs as follows:

SCUTE: to cool Liver fire and calm internal wind; it is used in many formulas for treating fire syndromes (inflammation and redness) and nervous problems; scute also harmonizes the Gallbladder which is the organ mediating Liver/Spleen interactions. Hence, when treating Liver Chi invading the Stomach/Spleen (e.g. for digestive disturbance, ulcer, nausea, food allergy, etc), bupleurum is combined with scute, and usually also with pinellia and ginger to treat the Stomach/Spleen disturbance.

PEONY: is said to soften the Liver and cool the Blood. It is used for hot flashes, sore throats (combined also with mentha), irritability, insomnia, and gynecologic problems. Peony is often employed in bupleurum when there is Blood deficiency. Scute is frequently included along with peony in the fire-purging formulas. Some persons, when taking a bupleurum harmonizing formula, will suddenly experience extreme anger or other emotional symptoms; in such cases, peony should be included in the formula. Tang-kuei is almost always included with peony to enhance the nourishing and activating of blood, and to relax tension.

CYPERUS: When Liver tension causes abdominal pain, menstrual irregularity, and bloating, bupleurum is often combined with cyperus. Bupleurum and cyperus are said to disperse stagnant Chi of the abdomen. Other aromatics are combined with bupleurum and cyperus, most often citrus, Chih-shih, Chih-ko, cardamon, and saussurea. Bupleurum and cyperus are used in the treatment of ulcer in persons of weak constitution, especially when combined with saussurea and cardamon.

CAUTIONS REGARDING THE USE OF BUPLEURUM FORMULAS

1) Because bupleurum dredges and disperses Chi, it can have a drying effect. Persons with deficiency of Blood and/or Yin should be given the appropriate tonics at the same time. Many bupleurum formulas already contain blood tonics.

2) Because bupleurum aids the rise of Chi, persons who tend to get headaches, nose bleeds, or other signs of flushing up of Chi should be given herbs that aid the descending of Chi, such as dragon bone and oyster shell, cinnamon plus rhubarb or coptis, cuscuta and rehmannia, etc.

Note: *In the following formula listings, ginger is indicated as "ganjiang," that is, dried ginger. In fact, several formulas would normally call for fresh ginger in making the teas. However, it is common for many herbalists to utilize the more convenient dried ginger, and in making the extract granules, the properties characteristic of dry ginger arise. In making herb teas, fresh ginger is considered to be more suitable for promoting surface circulation and dry ginger more suitable for internal circulation.*

小柴胡湯

MINOR BUPLEURUM COMBINATION

Xiao Chai Hu Tang

THERAPEUTIC PRINCIPLES: relieve Liver, harmonize Liver and Spleen, harmonize surface and interior.

INDICATIONS: subcostal bloating, intercostal neuralgia, weak digestion, nervousness, irritability, bitter taste in the mouth, hepatitis (acute or chronic), gallbladder disorders, ulcer, tendency to diarrhea, general weakness, prolonged cold/flu, combination of cold/flu with chronic disorder of Liver/Gallbladder (LV/GB) or Stomach/Spleen (ST/SP).

PULSE: tense, somewhat rapid, but not strong

TONGUE: moist; thin white tongue coating or no coating

HERBS AND ACTIONS: Bupleurum and scute relieve the Liver; ginseng, jujube, and licorice strengthen the Spleen; pinellia and ginger normalize digestive function and dry dampness and phlegm; bupleurum harmonizes interior and surface; ginger, jujube, and licorice normalize digestion and aid treatment of acute conditions.

TYPICAL MODIFICATIONS: For Kidney weakness, lower abdominal bloating, morning diarrhea, chronic yeast infections, and thirst, add hoelen, alisma, disocorea, and cuscuta; for abdominal pain, add cardamon and saussurea; for menstrual irregularity and pre-menstrual tension, add cyperus and peony; for Lung weakness and low resistance, add schizandra and astragalus; for recurrent Lung heat ailments, add coptis and trichosanthes seed (this will produce **Bupleurum and Scute Combination**), and if there is productive cough, use trichosanthes seed with platycodon and chih-shih (this will produce **Bupleurum, Chih-shih, and Platycodon Combination** with jujube added) or add platycodon and gypsum (this will produce **Bupleurum, Platycodon, and Gypsum Combination**); for dry cough, add ophiopogon and bamboo (this will produce **Ginseng and Bamboo Leaves Combination**); for stomach upset, edema, and severe thirst, add **Hoelen Five Herb Formula** (this will produce **Bupleurum and Hoelen Combination**); For muscle tension and for chronic intestinal disorders, add cinnamon twig and peony (this will produce **Bupleurum and Cinnamon Combination**); for pleurisy and wasting diseases involving the lungs, add chin-chiu, lycium bark, aster, tang-kuei, and mume (this will produce **Chin-chiu and Bupleurum Combination** with tortoise shell deleted).

7.0 Bupleurum	Chaihu	LV/GB; disperses Chi,
3.0 Scute	huangqin	purges fire
3.0 Ginseng	Renshen	SP/ST; tonifies Chi
2.0 Licorice	Gancao	
3.0 Jujube	Dazao	
5.0 Pinellia	Banxia	SP/ST; normalizes functions
2.0 Ginger	Shengjiang	

NOTES:

柴胡桂枝湯

BUPLEURUM AND CINNAMON COMBINATION

Chai Hu Gui Zhi Tang

THERAPEUTIC ACTIONS: relieve the Liver, relieve surface tension, harmonize Liver, Spleen, and Intestines, harmonize surface and interior.

INDICATIONS: chiropractic disorders (repeated loss of spinal alignment due to muscular tension), cold or flu in persons with internal disorder (Liver, Spleen, or Intestine disturbances), ulcer, subcostal pain, minor joint pain, headaches, hepatitis, Gallbladder disorders, chronic intestinal disorders, tension of abdominal muscles, epigastric fullness.

PULSE: floating, somewhat tense, or weak

TONGUE: white tongue coating

HERBS AND ACTIONS: Bupleurum, scute, and peony relieve the Liver; and in combination with cinnamon twig, relieve muscular tension; ginseng, jujube, and licorice strengthen the Spleen; ginger and pinellia normalize digestive functions; ginger, jujube, and licorice aid treatment of acute symptoms.

TYPICAL VARIATIONS: For shoulder/neck tension (including whiplash injury) add a large dose of pueraria; for arthritis, add coix and tang-kuei; for headaches, add chrysanthemum; for intestinal disorder with tendency to diarrhea, add hoelen and atractylodes; for cold or flu with headache, add schizonepeta and cnidium. For constipation, may add rhubarb.

5.0 Bupleurum	Chaihu	LV/GB; disperses Chi, purges fire
2.0 Scute	Huangqin	

BUPLEURUM AND CINNAMON COMBINATION

2.0 Ginseng	Renshen	SP/ST; tonifies Chi
1.5 Licorice	Gancao	
2.0 Jujube	Dazao	
4.0 Pinellia	Banxia	SP/ST; normalizes functions
1.0 Ginger	Shengjiang	
2.5 Cinnamon	Guizhi	LV; relaxes muscles,
2.5 Peony	Baishao	activates Blood

NOTES:

柴胡疏肝湯

BUPLEURUM AND CYPERUS COMBINATION

Chai Hu Shu Gan Tang

LITERAL: Bupleurum Smoothes the Liver Decoction

THERAPEUTIC PRINCIPLES: relieve the Liver, dispel stagnant Chi, purge the Gallbladder, promote Blood circulation.

INDICATIONS: cold hands and feet, fatigue, depression, gallbladder problems, pre-menstrual tension, nervousness and anxiety, irritability.

PULSE: tense, sinking

TONGUE: may have purple spots

HERBS AND ACTIONS: This formula is derived from Bupleurum and Chih-shih Formula, with blue citrus, cyperus, and cnidium added. Bupleurum, peony, and cyperus relieve the Liver and with blue citrus and chih-shih dispel stagnant Chi and purge the Gallbladder; peony and cnidium circulate the Blood; licorice is harmonizer.

TYPICAL VARIATIONS: For Blood stasis, add persica and carthamus; for abdominal pain, add corydalis and melia; for uterine tumor, add achyranthes, zedoria, moutan, and salvia; for Yin deficiency, add cooked rehmannia and alisma; for weak Spleen, add codonopsis, ginger and jujube; for anemia, add tang-kuei; for constipation, add gardenia; for ulcer, add pinellia, scute, and ginger; for chronic vaginal infection, add saussurea and gentiana.

4.0 Bupleurum	Chaihu	LV/GB; disperses Chi
3.0 Cyperus	Xiangfu	
2.0 Blue Citrus	Qingpi	
3.0 Chih-shih	Zhishi	

BUPLEURUM AND CYPERUS COMBINATION

4.0 Peony	Baishao	LV; activates Blood
3.0 Cnidium	Chuanxiong	
2.0 Licorice	Gancao	servant

NOTES:

柴胡桂枝乾姜湯

BUPLEURUM, CINNAMON, AND GINGER COMBINATION

Chai Hu Gui Zhi Gan Jiang Tang

THERAPEUTIC PRINCIPLES: clears heat, astringes sweating, moistens Lung, relieves flushing up.

INDICATIONS: fever, sweating, thirst, dry cough, heart palpitation, chest distress, chills in the limbs, acute bronchitis, hepatitis, and gallstones.

PULSE: fast, thin, or irregular

TONGUE: swollen, coated

HERBS AND ACTIONS: Bupleurum and scute relieve the Liver; oyster shell astringes sweating and reduces heart palpitation; trichosanthes root moistens the Lung; cinnamon twig relieves flushing up, ginger and licorice are harmonizers.

TYPICAL VARIATIONS: For muscle tension add peony and pueraria; for diarrhea or soft stools, add ginseng and hoelen; for cough with thick colored phlegm, add coptis; for hepatitis, add capillaris and chih-shih; for chronic bronchitis, add ginseng and jujube (this will produce **Bupleurum and Trichosanthes Root Combination** with oyster shell and cinnamon added).

6.0 Bupleurum	Chaihu	LV/GB; disperses Chi,
3.0 Scute	Huangqin	purges fire
3.0 Cinnamon	Guizhi	LU; activates surface
2.0 Ginger	Ganjiang	circulation
3.0 Oystershell	Muli	HT; reduces excessive sweating

3.0 Trichosanthes	Tianhuafen	LU; moistens lungs
2.0 Licorice	Gancao	servant

NOTES:

淨腑湯

BUPLEURUM AND PINELLIA COMBINATION

Jing Fu Tang

LITERAL: Clean the Hollow Organs Decoction

THERAPEUTIC PRINCIPLES: activate Blood, clear Moisture, strengthen Stomach and Spleen function.

INDICATIONS: tumors or hard masses in the abdomen, blockage and swelling of the hollow organs, peritonitis

PULSE: congested

TONGUE: may be moist or dry, coated

HERBS AND ACTIONS: This formula is made from **Bupleurum and Hoelen Combination** with scirpus, zedoria, and crataegus added to activate circulation of Blood and coptis added to purge fire. **Bupleurum and Hoelen Combination** is in turn made from Hoelen Five Herb Formula, which clears moisture and **Minor Bupleurum Combination** which disperses stagnant Liver Chi and normalizes Stomach/Spleen functions.

TYPICAL VARIATIONS: This is a large **Ming Dynasty formula** and is usually not modified. For more severe Blood stasis, add salvia and red peony; for phlegm obstruction, add bamboo and fritillaria; for irritability and tension, add peony; for anti-tumor activity, add hedyotis and coix.

3.0 Bupleurum	Chaihu	LV/GB; disperses Chi, purges fire
1.5 Scute	Huangqin	
1.0 Coptis	Huanglian	
3.0 Hoelen	Fuling	SP/KI; clears Moisture
1.5 Alisma	Zexie	
1.5 Polyporus	Zhuling	

BUPLEURUM AND PINELLIA COMBINATION

1.5 Ginseng	Renshen	SP; tonifies Chi
1.5 Atractylodes	Baizhu	
1.0 Licorice	Gancao	
1.0 Jujube	Dacao	
1.5 Scirpus	Sanling	LV; activates Blood
1.5 Zedoria	Erzhu	
2.0 Pinellia	Banxia	SP/ST; clears congestion
1.5 Crataegus	Shansha	
1.0 Ginger	Ganjiang	

NOTES:

柴胡加龍骨牡蠣湯

BUPLEURUM AND DRAGON BONE COMBINATION

Chai Hu Mu Li Lung Gu Tang

THERAPEUTIC PRINCIPLES: relieve the Liver, stabilize Shen, strengthen Spleen, normalize digestion, and purge the Colon and Gallbladder.

INDICATIONS: nervousness, irritability, insomnia, fatigue, depression, ulcer, neck and shoulder tension; digestive disturbance (flatulence, food allergy, stomachache, constipation), subcostal pressure and bloating, gallbladder disorders, epilepsy, twitching, jaw tension, headaches, unexpressed anger, drug withdrawal syndrome (nicotine, caffeine, valium, etc.).

PULSE: tense and fast; may be sinking and strong, or floating

TONGUE: tends to be reddish, tends to have yellow coating, especially towards back (may have no coating).

HERBS AND ACTIONS: Bupleurum and scute relieve the Liver; ginseng and jujube strengthen the Spleen; pinellia and ginger resolve digestive disturbance; hoelen, dragon bone, and oyster shell stabilize the Shen; cinnamon with rhubarb relieves flushing up of Chi; rhubarb purges the Large Intestine and with bupleurum and scute purges the Gallbladder.

TYPICAL MODIFICATIONS: For emotional disturbance, insomnia, and vivid dreaming, add zizyphus, biota, and polygala; for shoulder/neck tension, add pueraria; for hypertension and tension headaches, add gambir and chrysanthemum; for depression, add chih-ko and cyperus; for abdominal bloating, add magnolia bark and atractylodes; for Lung heat and thirst, add trichosanthes root; for nightsweats, add moutan and rehmannia.

BUPLEURUM AND DRAGON BONE COMBINATION

5.0 Bupleurum	Chaihu	LV/GB; disperses Chi,
2.5 Scute	Huangqin	purges fire
2.5 Ginseng	Renshen	SP/ST; tonifies Chi
2.5 Jujube	Dazao	
4.0 Pinellia	Banxia	SP/ST; normalizes functions
2.0 Ginger	Ganjiang	
2.5 Dragon bone	Lunggu	HT; sedates Shen
2.5 Oyster shell	Muli	
3.0 Hoelen	Fuling	
1.0 Rhubarb	Dahuang	relieves flushing up
3.0 Cinnamon	Guizhi	

NOTES:

大柴胡湯

MAJOR BUPLEURUM COMBINATION

Da Chai Hu Tang

THERAPEUTIC PRINCIPLES: relieve the Liver, purge the Gallbladder and Large Intestine, harmonize Liver/Spleen.

INDICATIONS: gallbladder disorders, hepatitis, constipation, abdominal bloating, severe chest distress, indigestion, food allergy, obesity, hypertension, late onset diabetes, subcostal pressure, nervousness, irritability, insomnia.

PULSE: strong, sinking

TONGUE: tends to red; thick white fur or yellow to grey coating which may be greasy

HERBS AND ACTIONS: Bupleurum, scute, and peony relieve the Liver; rhubarb and Chih-shih purge the Gallbladder and Large Intestine; pinellia, ginger, and jujube normalize digestive function.

TYPICAL VARIATIONS: For Yin deficiency add alisma, cornus, and lycium; for digestive weakness, add codonopsis and licorice; for more severe constipation, add mirabilitum and licorice; for flatulence, add magnolia bark and cardamon; for pain of the liver and gallbladder, add corydalis; for insomnia, add hoelen, dragon bone, and oyster shell; for gallstones or jaundice, add capillaris and gardenia; for inflammation of the throat, mouth, or lips, add bamboo leaf and forsythia.

6.0 Bupleurum	Chaihu	LV/GB; disperses Chi,
3.0 Scute	Huangqin	purges fire
3.0 Peony	Baishou	
3.0 Pinellia	Banxia	SP/ST; normalizes functions
4.0 Ginger	Ganjiang	

MAJOR BUPLEURUM COMBINATION

1.0 Rhubarb	Dahuang	SP/ST; purges accumulation
2.0 Chih-shih	Zhishi	
3.0 Jujube	Dazao	servant; moderates purgative

NOTES:

柴葛解肌湯

BUPLEURUM AND PUERARIA COMBINATION

Chai Ge Jie Ji Tang

LITERAL: Bupleurum and Pueraria Relieve the Muscles Decoction

THERAPEUTIC PRINCIPLES: dispel wind, relieve the Liver, relieve surface tension.

INDICATIONS: shoulder/neck tension, headache and general body aches; Lung heat ailments (including pneumonia), thirst.

PULSE: fast, broad, floating

TONGUE: may be red, may have yellow coating

HERBS AND ACTIONS: Bupleurum, scute, and peony relieve the Liver; chiang-huo, angelica, and pueraria dispel wind in the Upper Warmer, relax muscle tension, and relieve pain; gypsum and platycodon treat Lung heat and swollen glands; ginger, jujube, and licorice aid treatment of acute conditions.

TYPICAL VARIATIONS: This is a large **Ming Dynasty formula;** it is usually not modified; for sinus congestion add ma-huang and magnolia flower; for headache, add vitex, cnidium, and chrysanthemum; for chronic Lung heat, add morus bark; for pain in the limbs and joints, add arisaema and bamboo sap; for sore throat, add mentha and chih-ko.

4.0 Bupleurum	Chaihu	LV/GB; disperses Chi, purges fire
3.0 Scute	Huangqin	
3.0 Peony	Baishao	
4.0 Pueraria	Gegen	LU; dispels wind, relieves pain
2.0 Chiang-huo	Qianghuo	
2.0 Angelica	Baizhi	

2.0 Platycodon	Jiegeng	LU; relieves inflammation
5.0 Gypsum	Shigao	
1.0 Ginger	Ganjiang	servants
2.0 Licorice	Gancao	
2.0 Jujube	Dazao	

NOTES:

柴胡清肝湯

BUPLEURUM AND REHMANNIA COMBINATION

Chai Hu Qing Gan Tang

LITERAL: Bupleurum Clear the Liver Decoction

THERAPEUTIC PRINCIPLES: purge fire, nourish Blood, relieve surface heat, relieve the Liver.

INDICATIONS: swollen lymph glands, sore throat, skin eruptions, headaches, red eyes, spontaneous bleeding.

PULSE: tense, floating, fast

TONGUE: red, may have no coating or thin yellow coating

HERBS AND ACTIONS: This formula is made from **Tang-kuei and Gardenia Combination** which nourishes Liver Blood and purges Liver fire to treat skin disorders and spontaneous bleeding, by adding bupleurum and peony to relieve Liver tension, forsythia to clean toxins, and the combination of trichosanthes root, platycodon, mentha, and arctium to resolve inflammation, phlegm congestion, and itching.

TYPICAL VARIATIONS: This is a large **Ming Dynasty formula** that is usually not modified; for deficiency fire, add anemarrhena; for headache, add chrysanthemum or vitex; for sores in the mouth or menopausal hot flashes, add moutan and chih-ko; for thirst, add gypsum; for mouth sores, add moutan and scrophularia; for spontaneous bleeding, add artemesia and gelatin.

2.0 Bupleurum	Chaihu	LV/GB; disperses Chi,
1.5 Scute	Huangqin	purges fire
1.5 Tang-kuei	Danggui	LV; nourishes and
1.5 Peony	Baishao	activates Blood
1.5 Cnidium	Chuanziong	
1.5 Rehmannia	Dihuang	

BUPLEURUM AND REHMANNIA COMBINATION

1.5 Coptis	Huanglian	LV/HT; purges fire,
1.5 Phellodendron	Huangbai	dries dampness
1.5 Gardenia	Zhizi	
1.5 Forsythia	Lianqiao	
1.5 Mentha	Bohe	LU; clears surface heat
1.5 Arctium	Niubangzi	
1.5 Platycodon	Jiegeng	LU; clears phlegm and pus
1.5 Trichosanthes	Tianhuafen	
1.5 Licorice	Gancao	servant

NOTES:

四逆散

BUPLEURUM AND CHIH-SHIH FORMULA

Si Ni San

LITERAL: Four Distressed Limbs Decoction

THERAPEUTIC PRINCIPLES: relieves the Liver.

INDICATIONS: cold hands and feet, spasms in the limbs, gallbladder disorders, abdominal pain and distension

PULSE: tight, floating, rapid

TONGUE: thin white coating or no coating

HERBS AND ACTIONS: Bupleurum and peony relieve the Liver; chih-shih disperses stagnant Chi and clears the gallbladder; licorice with peony relaxes abdominal muscle spasms.

TYPICAL VARIATIONS: For surface muscle spasms, add cinnamon twig; for facial flushing and headache, add mentha and chih-ko; for severe abdominal pain, add cyperus, blue citrus, and cnidium (this will produce **Bupleurum and Cyperus Combination**); for anemia, add Tang-kuei; for gastric ulcer, add ginseng and ginger; for edema, add areca seed, tortoise shell, and atractylodes (this will produce **Bupleurum and Tortoise Shell Combination**); for abdominal tension and fullness, add scute, rhubarb, pinellia, and ginger (this will produce **Major Bupleurum Combination** with licorice replacing jujube).

5.0 Bupleurum	Chaihu	LV/GB; relieves tension
4.0 Peony	Baishao	
2.0 Chih-shih	Zhishi	SP/ST; clears accumulation
1.5 Licorice	Gancao	servant

NOTES:

竹如温膽湯

BAMBOO AND GINSENG COMBINATION

Chu Ru Wen Dan Tang

LITERAL: Bamboo Warm the Gallbladder Decoction

THERAPEUTIC PRINCIPLES: relieve the Liver, disperses stagnant Chi, relieve Lung heat, dissolve heated sputum, harmonize interior and surface, clear phlegm congestion of the orifices of the Heart.

INDICATIONS: mental distress and insomnia related to excessive sputum disease; prolonged febrile disease, facial flushing, restlessness, absent-mindedness, nightmares, copious sputum, swollen glands, alcoholism, neurosis, swelling or numbness of the arms.

PULSE: fast, congested or slippery

TONGUE: greasy coating

HERBS AND ACTIONS: This formula is made from **Citrus and Pinellia Combination** by adding Chi-dispersing and Shen-sedating herbs. Pinellia, citrus, and ginger dissolve phlegm, and with bamboo, platycodon, and chih-shih, dissolve heated phlegm; bupleurum and cyperus relieve the Liver and with citrus and chih-shih, disperse stagnant Chi and purge the Gallbladder; coptis, platycodon, bupleurum, and bamboo relieve heat in the chest; ginseng, hoelen, ginger, and licorice strengthen the Spleen and Heart.

TYPICAL VARIATIONS: This is a large **Ming Dynasty formula;** it is usually not modified; for insomnia, add zizyphus and biota; for constipation add gardenia; for severe mental distress and thirst, add ophiopogon and gypsum; for severe cough, add trichosanthes seed and eriobotrya; for excessive thick sputum, add fritillaria and morus.

BAMBOO AND GINSENG COMBINATION

5.0 Bupleurum	Chaihu	LV/GB; disperses Chi
2.0 Cyperus	Xiangfu	
1.0 Chih-shih	Zhishi	SP; clears congestion
1.0 Citrus	Chenpi	and stagnation
3.0 Platycodon	Jiegeng	LU; clears phlegm
3.0 Bamboo	Zhuru	
3.0 Pinellia	Banxia	SP/ST; normalizes functions
1.0 Ginger	Ganjiang	
2.0 Coptis	Huanglian	HT; purges fire, sedates Shen
3.0 Hoelen	Fuling	
2.0 Ginseng	Renshen	SP; tonifies Chi
1.0 Licorice	Gancao	

Note: *Pinellia plus citrus is said to "warm the gallbladder," treating phlegm that arises from incomplete digestion of fats.*

NOTES:

加味逍遥散

BUPLEURUM AND PEONY FORMULA

Jia Wei Xiao Yao San

LITERAL: Added Flavors Freedom Powder

THERAPEUTIC PRINCIPLES: relieve Liver, nourish Blood, relieve Blood heat and Upper Warmer surface heat, dispel damp-heat of Lower Warmer.

INDICATIONS: pre-menstrual tension, menopausal hot flashes, insomnia, fatigue, constipation, pale complexion, menstrual irregularities, chronic or recurrent vaginal infections, dysmenorrhea, liver cirrhosis, tendonitis, bitter taste in the mouth.

PULSE: tense, somewhat hollow; may be fast

TONGUE: pale tongue, small cracks, thin coating

HERBS AND ACTIONS: This formula is derived from **Bupleurum and Tang-kuei Formula,** by adding moutan and gardenia; it is also derived from **Gardenia and Hoelen Formula,** which is used to treat Lower Warmer heat, by adding Liver and Spleen active herbs. Bupleurum with peony relieves the Liver, with gardenia purges the Gallbladder, and with mentha relieves surface heat of the Upper Warmer; gardenia, peony, and moutan relieve Blood heat and abdominal pain; ginger, licorice, hoelen, and atractylodes strengthen the Stomach/Spleen and with gardenia relieve damp-heat of the Lower Warmer; tang-kuei and peony nourish and circulate the Blood.

TYPICAL VARIATIONS: For menstrual irregularity and pain, add cyperus and persica; for weak Spleen, add codonopsis and jujube; for insomnia, add dragon bone and oyster shell; for Yin deficiency, add cooked rehmannia and alisma or add eclipta and ligustrum; for abdominal bloating, add citrus and magnolia bark; for acne, add arctium and forsythia; for tendency to diarrhea, add pinellia and dioscorea;

for menstrual headache, add schizonepeta and angelica; for gallstones, add chih-shih; for arthralgia, add cinnamon twig; for sore throat, add chih-ko; for nervous excitability, add gambir and cnidium; for tendonitis, add chaenomeles.

3.0 Bupleurum	Chaihu	LV; disperses Chi,
1.0 Mentha	Bohe	relieves surface heat
3.0 Tang-kuei	Danggui	LV; nourishes and
3.0 Peony	Baishao	activates Blood
3.0 Atractylodes	Baizhu	SP/ST; tonifies Chi,
3.0 Hoelen	Fuling	clears dampness
2.0 Gardenia	Zhizi	HT; purges fire, cools Blood
2.0 Moutan	Mudanpi	
1.0 Ginger	Ganjiang	servants
2.0 Licorice	Gancao	

NOTES:

抑肝散

BUPLEURUM FORMULA

Yi Gan San

LITERAL: Normalize the Liver Powder

THERAPEUTIC PRINCIPLES: relieve the Liver, nourish Blood, purge fire, and normalize the Stomach and Spleen.

INDICATIONS: irritability, insomnia, grinding of teeth, dizziness, heart palpitations, muscle spasms, hypertension.

PULSE: weak, rapid

TONGUE: stiff or quivering

HERBS AND ACTIONS: Bupleurum relieves the Liver and with gambir clears Liver heat that causes headaches and neurotic symptoms; tang-kuei and cnidium activate and nourish the Blood; hoelen and atractylodes normalize the Stomach and Spleen; licorice is harmonizer.

TYPICAL ADDITIONS: For gallbladder congestion causing digestive disturbance, phlegm congestion, and mental disturbances, add pinellia and citrus (this will produce **Bupleurum and Citrus, Pinellia Formula**); for more severe heat and tension, add peony and chih-shih; for headaches, add pueraria; for depression and menstrual disorders, add peony, mentha, and ginger (this will produce **Bupleurum and Tang-kuei Formula** with cnidium and gambir added).

2.0 Bupleurum	Chaihu	LV/GB; purges fire,
3.0 Gambir	Gouteng	relieves spasm
3.0 Tang-kuei	Danggui	LV; nourishes and
3.0 Cnidium	Chuanxiong	activates Blood
4.0 Hoelen	Fuling	SP/ST; moves Moisture
4.0 Atractylodes	Baizhu	
1.5 Licorice	Gancao	servant

柴胡厚朴湯

BUPLEURUM AND MAGNOLIA COMBINATION

Chai Hu Hou Pu Tang

THERAPEUTIC PRINCIPLES: disperses stagnant Chi, clears Moisture.

INDICATIONS: abdominal distention, edema, asthmatic breathing, fullness in the chest; heart palpitation, neurosis

PULSE: slippery or choppy

TONGUE: swollen, pale, white creamy coating or white thin coating.

HERBS AND ACTIONS: Bupleurum, magnolia bark, citrus, and perilla disperse stagnant Chi; hoelen and areca seed aid in clearing stagnant moisture.

TYPICAL MODIFICATIONS: For asthma, add Ma-huang, apricot seed, and licorice (these three make up **Ma-huang, Licorice and Apricot Seed Combination**; the combination then produces **Ma-huang and Magnolia Combination** with areca seed and hoelen added); for severe edema, add ginger and morus (this will produce **Hoelen and Areca Combination** with magnolia, bupleurum, and perilla added); for constipation, add chih-shih; for abdominal pain, add cyperus and aquilaria.

5.0 Bupleurum	Chaihu	LV; disperses Chi
1.5 Perilla	Zisuye	LU/SP; disperses congested Chi/Moisture
3.0 Magnolia bark	Houpo	
3.0 Citrus	Chenpi	
3.0 Areca seed	Bingliang	
5.0 Hoelen	Fuling	SP/ST; clears accumulated Moisture

升陽散火湯

BUPLEURUM AND GINSENG COMBINATION

Sheng Yang San Huo Tang

LITERAL: Raise the Yang and Disperse the Fire Decoction

THERAPEUTIC PRINCIPLES: relieve the Liver, tonify Chi, Blood and Yin, raise the Yang, purge fire, dispel sputum

INDICATIONS: chronic bronchitis, tightness of the chest, wheezing, pallor.

PULSE: tense, somewhat hollow or thin, rapid

TONGUE: white coating

HERBS AND ACTIONS: This formula is made from **Bupleurum and Tang-kuei Formula** by adding ginseng, citrus, ophiopogon, and scute. Citrus disperses stagnant Chi and sputum; ophiopogon clears heat while nourishing Yin; scute purges fire of the Liver and Lungs.

TYPICAL VARIATIONS: For thick phlegm, add fritillaria and bamboo; for asthmatic breathing, add morus and ginkgo; for shoulder/neck tension, add cinnamon twig.

4.0 Bupleurum	Chaihu	LV/GB; disperses Chi, purges fire
4.0 Scute		
3.0 Tang-kuei	Danggui	LV; tonifies Blood
3.0 Peony	Baishao	
3.0 Ginseng	Renshen	SP/ST; tonifies Chi
3.0 Atractylodes	Baizhu	
3.0 Citrus	Chenpi	SP/LU; clears Moisture, sputum
3.0 Hoelen		
4.0 Ophiopogon	Maimendong	LU; tonifies Yin

1.5 Ginger	Ganjiang	servants
1.5 Licorice	Gancao	

NOTES:

疏肝湯

BUPLEURUM AND EVODIA COMBINATION

Shu Gan Tang

LITERAL: Relieve the Liver Decoction

THERAPEUTIC PRINCIPLES: relieve the Liver, activate circulation of Chi and Blood, relieve pain in the Stomach and ribs.

PULSE: tense, knotty

TONGUE: purplish spots

HERBS AND ACTIONS: Bupleurum and peony relieve the Liver; Tang-kuei, cnidium, peony, persica, and carthamus activate Blood circulation; evodia and coptis relieve pain in the area of the Stomach that arises from Liver Chi stagnation; blue citrus and chih-ko disperse stagnant Chi.

TYPICAL VARIATIONS: For Chi weakness, add codonopsis and white atractylodes; for lower abdominal pain, add cyperus and moutan; for endometriosis add cinnamon and akebia; for digestive disturbance, add pinellia and ginger.

5.0 Bupleurum	Chaihu	LV/GB; purges fire
1.0 Coptis	Huanglian	
5.0 Tang-kuei	Danggui	LV; nourishes and activates Blood
3.0 Peony	Baishao	
3.0 Cnidium	Chuanxiong	
0.5 Evodia	Wuzhuyu	ST; disperses Chi
3.0 Blue citrus	Qingpi	
2.0 Chih-ko	Zhiqiao	
1.0 Carthamus	Honghua	LV; breaks up clots, activates Blood
3.0 Persica	Taoren	

BUPLEURUM AND EVODIA COMBINATION

Note: *The combination of evodia and coptis is also known as the "pill of left gold;" it is added to prescriptions for the treatment of Liver Chi invading the Stomach.*

NOTES:

INTRODUCTION TO GINSENG

Ginseng is the best known and most highly respected of Chinese herbs. Its uses in formulas are very diverse. When ginseng is a principal herb of the formula, the function of the combination is to enhance or normalize digestive processes and strengthen Chi. When it plays a secondary role, it usually protects the Chi from destruction either by the disease process or by the strong action of other herbs. It can also be used as a sedative in formulas for disturbances of the Spirit.

Typically, the person with a Chi problem has the following types of symptoms:

- weight problems
- food intolerance
- lethargy
- weakness of muscles
- pallor
- digestive disturbances
- eliminative disorders
- hernia or other prolapse
- emotional instability
- weak pulse
- swollen tongue

Long term digestive disorders can lead to weakness of the Lung energy, with allergies (such as hayfever) and frequent colds and flus. Further, there may develop autoimmune disorders, such as rheumatoid arthritis.

STANDARD MATCHING IN GINSENG FORMULAS

LICORICE: is nearly always used as a complementary Chi tonic. It enhances the actions of ginseng.

ATRACTYLODES: is a frequent companion to ginseng in formulas and is only deleted in some cases where its effects on drying internal moisture might be undesirable.

PINELLIA: whenever there is notable digestive disturbance, pinellia accompanies ginseng. With citrus it aids gallbladder function in digesting fats, and with ginger it settles nausea, vomiting, and diarrhea.

TANG-KUEI: when the Blood is weak, the Spleen may be strengthened with ginseng in order to produce Blood, and Tang-kuei (usually with peony) is added to further nourish the Blood.

ASTRAGALUS: for severe weakness, nightsweats, and immunologic disorders, astragalus is added to consolidate the surface, build up the Chi, and normalize the immune system functions.

CAUTIONS ABOUT GINSENG FORMULAS

Persons suffering from Blood heat, including spontaneous bleeding, insomnia, restlessness, and upper body inflammation, may experience a worsening of symptoms because ginseng, especially the Korean ginseng used in Sun Ten formulas, tends to heat the blood and aid the rising of Chi.

GINSENG VERSUS CODONOPSIS

In mainland China, virtually all formulas calling for ginseng are now prepared with the less expensive Chi tonic codonopsis. Codonopsis has a milder action, is less heating, and is best used for maintaining the Chi rather than for strongly restoring weakened digestive function and deficient Chi. Ginseng is combined with Kidney tonics to restore "original Chi."

四君子湯

FOUR MAJOR HERBS COMBINATION

Si Jun Zi Tang

THERAPEUTIC PRINCIPLES: tonify Chi, strengthen Spleen, move Moisture.

INDICATIONS: weak digestion, low body weight, tendency to diarrhea, anemia, fatigue, loss of appetite, cold limbs, difficulty getting up in the morning, sleepiness after meals.

PULSE: sinking, soft

TONGUE: pale, moist, may be swollen; no fur or thin white fur

HERBS AND ACTIONS: Ginseng, licorice, white atractylodes, and jujube are Chi tonics and with hoelen and ginger, they strengthen the Spleen; atractylodes and hoelen move Moisture.

TYPICAL VARIATIONS: For slippery pulse and gastric disturbance, add pinellia and citrus (this will produce **Six Major Herbs Combination**); for anemia (but no diarrhea), add **Tang-kuei Four Combination** (this will produce **Tang-kuei and Ginseng Eight Combination**); for hernia, prolapse of organs, and hemorrhoids, add astragalus, bupleurum, cimicifuga, citrus, and tang-kuei (this will produce **Ginseng and Astragalus Combination**); for acute gastric disturbance and ulcer, add pinellia, citrus, coptis, scute, and oyster shell (this will produce **Pinellia and Ginseng Six Combination**); for chronic gastric disturbance and ulcer, add dolichos, dioscorea, cardamon, lotus seed, platycodon, and coix (this will produce **Ginseng and Atractylodes Formula**); for chronic GI disturbance with pain, add cardamon, saussurea, cyperus, magnolia bark, and citrus (this will produce **Cyperus and Cluster Combination**); for indigestion, loss of appetite, and diarrhea, add lotus seed, dioscorea, crataegus, citrus, and alisma (this will produce **Lotus and Citrus Combination**); for summer heat syndrome with diarrhea, add pueraria, agasthache, and saussurea (this will produce **Atractylodes and Pueraria Formula**).

4.0 Ginseng	Renshen	SP; tonifies Chi
1.5 Licorice	Gancao	
4.0 Atractylodes	Baizhu	SP/ST; clears Moisture
4.0 Hoelen	Fuling	

Note: *Ginger and jujube are sometimes added as servants.*

NOTES:

六君子湯

SIX MAJOR HERBS COMBINATION

Liu Jun Zi Tang

THERAPEUTIC PRINCIPLES: tonify Chi, strengthen spleen, normalize stomach function.

INDICATIONS: nausea, vomiting, phlegm production, indigestion, diarrhea.

PULSE: sinking, slippery

TONGUE: coated, may be greasy

HERBS AND ACTIONS: This formula is derived from **Four Major Herbs Combination** by adding pinellia and citrus, which clear phlegm, and remove accumulation of the ST and/or SP, and ginger and licorice to further normalize digestive processes.

TYPICAL VARIATIONS: For severe indigestion with diarrhea, add dioscorea, lotus seed, crataegus, and alisma (this will produce **Lotus and Citrus Combination** with pinellia added); for intestinal parasites, add mume, agastache, magnolia bark, and tsao-kao (this will produce **Ginseng Stomach Combination**); for weakness with gastric ulcer, add bupleurum and peony (this will produce **B.P. and Six Major Herb Combination**); for abdominal pain due to gastric disturbance, add saussurea and cardamon (this will produce **Saussurea and Cardamon Combination**); for chronic weakness and for hernia or other prolapse, add bupleurum, cimicifuga, astragalus, and tang-kuei (this will produce **Ginseng and Astragalus Combination** with pinellia added); for heartburn and intestinal gas, add coptis, scute, and oyster shell (this will produce **Pinellia and Ginseng Six Combination**); for nausea with tiredness and bloating after meals, add shen-chu, malt, cardamon, and crataegus (this will produce Cardamon and **Six Major Herbs Combination**); for acute gastro-intestinal disorder with diarrhea, add magnolia bark and agastache (this will produce **Pinellia, Atractylodes, and Agastache Formula** with ginseng and hoelen added).

4.0 Ginseng	Renshen	SP; tonifies Chi
1.0 Licorice	Gancao	
2.0 Jujube	Dacao	
4.0 Atractylodes	Baizhu	SP/ST; clears Moisture
4.0 Hoelen	Fuling	
4.0 Pinellia	Banxia	SP/ST; normalizes functions
2.0 Citrus	Chenpi	
2.0 Ginger	Ganjiang	

NOTES:

十全大補湯

GINSENG AND TANG-KUEI TEN COMBINATION

Shi Quan Da Bu Tang

LITERAL: Ten Herb Complete and Great Tonifying Decoction

THERAPEUTIC PRINCIPLES: nourish Blood, tonify Chi, strengthen Spleen.

INDICATIONS: general debility, anemia, sinking Chi, low body weight, loss of appetite, slight bloating, weak musculature, chronic dry skin disorders, weakness of the knees, recovery from surgery, injury, or childbirth.

PULSE: weak

TONGUE: pale, small amount of white fur or no fur

HERBS AND ACTIONS: The formula is derived from **Four Major Herbs Combination** plus **Tang-kuei Four Combination** (together forming **Tang-kuei and Ginseng Eight Combination**), with cinnamon bark and astragalus added. Ginseng, astragalus, licorice, and white atractylodes are Chi tonics and with hoelen strengthen the Spleen; tang-kuei, peony, cnidium, and rehmannia nourish the Blood; cinnamon bark dispels chills and supplements Yang.

TYPICAL VARIATIONS: For sinking Chi, add bupleurum and cimicifuga; for insomnia and emotional disturbance, add longan, zizyphus, and polygala; for weak Lung Chi, add schizandra; for night sweats, increase the amount of astragalus and add cuscuta; for chronic skin disorders, add coix; for reduced function of all organs, add schizandra, polygala, and citrus (this will produce **Ginseng Nutritive Combination** with cnidium added); for spinal cord inflammation and low back pain, add eucommia, anemarrhena, and phellodendron.

GINSENG AND TANG-KUEI TEN COMBINATION

3.0 Ginseng	Renshen	SP; tonifies Chi
1.0 Licorice	Gancao	
3.0 Astragalus	Huangqi	
3.0 Atractylodes	Baizhu	SP/ST; dispels Moisture
3.0 Hoelen	Fuling	
3.0 Tang-kuei	Danggui	LV; nourishes Blood
3.0 Peony	Baishao	
3.0 Cnidium	Chuanxiong	
3.0 Rehmannia	Dihuang	
3.0 Cinnamon bark	Rougui	KI; tonifies Yang

NOTES:

半夏瀉心湯

PINELLIA COMBINATION

Ban Xia Xie Xin Tang

LITERAL: Pinellia Purge the Heart Decoction

THERAPEUTIC PRINCIPLES: normalize digestive function, dry dampness, dispel "water toxin," relieve nausea, purge Heart fire.

INDICATIONS: nausea, vomiting, diarrhea, ulcer

PULSE: fast, slippery

TONGUE: greasy coating

HERBS AND ACTIONS: Pinellia and ginger normalize digestive function; ginseng, licorice, and jujube strengthen Stomach/Spleen; coptis and scute purge Heart fire, relieve gastro-intestinal infection, and reduce inflammation.

TYPICAL VARIATIONS: For Liver tension, add bupleurum (this will produce **Minor Bupleurum Combination** with coptis added); for stomach pain, add cardamon and saussurea; for chronic diarrhea, add pueraria; for halitosis, increase the amount of ginger; for sense of lump in the throat, add magnolia bark; for chest distension, add bupleurum and trichosanthes seed (this will produce **Bupleurum and Scute Combination**); for acute gastric disturbance, add cinnamon (this will produce **Coptis Combination** with scute added); for halitosis, cramping, and borborgmus, increase the amount of ginger (this will produce **Pinellia and Ginger Combination**).

3.0 Ginseng	Renshen	SP; tonifies Chi
3.0 Jujube	Dazao	
3.0 Licorice	Gancao	
3.0 Scute	Huangqin	LV/HT; purges fire
3.0 Coptis	Huanglian	

PINELLIA COMBINATION

6.0 Pinellia	Banxia	SP/ST; normalizes functions
3.0 Ginger	Ganjiang	

NOTES:

大防風湯

MAJOR SILER COMBINATION

Da Fang Feng Tang

THERAPEUTIC PRINCIPLES: tonify Chi, Yang, and Blood, and dispel wind.

INDICATIONS: arthritis, myelitis.

PULSE: deep, thin

TONGUE: swollen, pale

HERBS AND ACTIONS: This formula is made from **Ginger and Tang-kuei Ten Combination** by adding astragalus, eucommia, achyranthes, siler, and chiang-huo (however, cinnamon bark is replaced here by aconite, and hoelen is replaced by ginger). Eucommia and aconite serve as Yang tonics; siler and chiang-huo dispel wind; achyranthes strengthens the lower body and promotes Blood circulation; astragalus improves the Chi tonification and Blood nourishing properties of the formula; ginger, jujube, and licorice are servants.

TYPICAL VARIATIONS: This is a large **Ming Dynasty formula,** and is usually not modified; for edema, add atractylodes, hoelen, and alisma; for greater Yang tonification, add dipsacus; for strong Blood activation, add carthamus.

1.5 Ginseng	Renshen	SP: tonifies Chi
3.0 Atractylodes	Baizhu	
3.0 Astragalus	Huangqi	
1.5 Licorice	Gancao	
1.5 Jujube	Dazao	
3.0 Tang-kuei	Danggui	LV; nourishes and activates Blood
3.0 Peony	Baishao	
3.0 Cnidium	Chuanqiong	
3.0 Rehmannia	Dihuang	
1.5 Achyranthes	Niuxi	

MAJOR SILER COMBINATION

3.0 Eucommia	Duzhong	KI; tonifies Yang
1.0 Aconite	Fuzi	
3.0 Siler	Fangfeng	LU; dispels wind
1.5 Chiang-huo	Qianghuo	
1.5 Ginger	Ganjiang	

NOTES:

人參養榮湯

GINSENG NUTRITIVE COMBINATION

Ren Shen Yang Yung Tang

LITERAL TRANSLATION: Ginseng Nourish the Impaired Decoction

THERAPEUTIC PRINCIPLES: tonify Chi, nourish Blood, supplement Yang, strengthen all organ systems.

INDICATIONS: general debility, low body weight, nightsweats, insomnia, loss of hair, pale complexion, loss of appetite, fatigue, asthma.

PULSE: weak

TONGUE: pale, little coating

HERBS AND ACTIONS: The base of this formula is **Ginseng and Tang-kuei Ten Combination,** which tonifies Spleen Chi, nourishes the Blood, and supplements Yang (only cnidium is deleted from the formula); polygala, which strengthens the Heart and Kidney; schizandra, which strengthens the Lung and Kidney; and citrus, which dispels stagnant Chi, are added.

TYPICAL VARIATIONS: For invasion of wind producing headaches, skin eruptions, or infections, add siler and schizonepeta; for Lung tonification, add platycodon; for Heart tonification, add longan; for enhancing Stomach/Spleen functions, add dioscorea and crataegus; for sinking Chi, add bupleurum and cimicifuga; for nightsweats, add oyster shell; for low back ache, add eucommia; for numbness and pain of the legs, add achyranthes, chin-chiu, siler, and chiang-huo; for insomnia and heart palpitations, add zizyphus and biota; for abdominal bloating, add magnolia bark and chaenomeles.

GINSENG NUTRITIVE COMBINATION

3.0 Ginseng	Renshen	SP; tonifies Chi
1.5 Licorice	Gancao	
2.5 Astragalus	Huangqi	
4.0 Atractylodes	Baizhu	
4.0 Tang-kuei	Danggui	LV; nourishes Blood
4.0 Peony	Baishao	
4.0 Rehmannia	Dihuang	
2.5 Cinnamon bark	Rougui	KI; strengthens Kidney
1.5 Polygala	Yuanzhi	
1.5 Schizandra	Wuweizi	
4.0 Hoelen	Fuling	
2.5 Citrus	Chenpi	servant; disperses Chi

NOTES:

歸脾湯

GINSENG AND LONGAN COMBINATION

Gui Pi Tang

LITERAL: Restoring the Spleen Decoction

THERAPEUTIC PRINCIPLES: strengthen the Spleen and Heart, tonify Chi, nourish Blood, stabilize Shen.

INDICATIONS: anemia, insomnia, immune system weakness, nightsweats, general weakness, heart palpitations, loss of memory, excessive worry, neurotic symptoms, fatigue, hemorrhaging.

PULSE: weak

TONGUE: pale, no tongue fur

HERBS AND ACTIONS: The formula is derived from **Four Major Herbs Combination** to strengthen the Spleen and tonify Chi; this is supplemented by tang-kuei and longan to nourish the Blood; polygala, zizyphus, and longan to nourish the Heart and stabilize the Shen, and saussurea to dispel stagnant Chi.

TYPICAL VARIATIONS: For additional sedative action, add biota; for flushing up, add cinnamon bark; for weakness in the lower body, add achyranthes and ho-shou-wu; for chronic yeast infection, add dioscorea and gardenia; for Liver tension and constipation, add bupleurum and gardenia (this will produce **Ginseng, Bupleurum, and Longan Combination**); for Blood stasis in the Lower Warmer, add cnidium, achyranthes, and moutan; for sinking Chi add bupleurum and cimicifuga; for anemia, add cnidium and peony; for chronic cough, add schizandra and pinellia; for excessive menstrual bleeding, add artemesia and gelatin; for excessive sweating and fatigue, add astragalus.

GINSENG AND LONGAN COMBINATION

3.0 Ginseng	Renshen	SP; tonifies Chi
1.0 Licorice	Gancao	
2.0 Astragalus	Huangqi	
3.0 Hoelen	Fuling	ST/SP; disperses dampness
3.0 Atractylodes	Baizhu	
2.0 Tang-kuei	Danggui	HT; nurtures Heart, pacifies Spirit
1.0 Polygala	Yuanzhi	
3.0 Longan	Longyanrou	
3.0 Zizyphus	Suanzaoren	
1.0 Saussurea	Muxiang	SP/LV; disperses Chi
1.0 Ginger	Ganjiang	servants
1.0 Jujube	Dazao	

NOTES:

天王補心丹

GINSENG AND ZIZYPHUS FORMULA

Tien Wang Bu Xin Dan

LITERAL: Heavenly Ruler's Nourish the Heart Elixir

THERAPEUTIC PRINCIPLES: nourish the heart, sedate spirit, disperse phlegm congestion of the orifices, dispel stagnant Blood.

INDICATIONS: insomnia, vivid dreaming, amnesia, mental dysfunction, emotional instability, heart palpitation.

PULSE: rapid, thin, congested

TONGUE: red, no coating or thin greasy coating

HERBS AND ACTIONS: Ophiopogon, scrophularia, rehmannia, biotia, and zizyphus nourish the Heart; acorus, biota, platycodon, and polygala disperse phlegm congestion of the orifices and calm the spirit; coptis purges Heart fire; ginseng, hoelen, and schizandra are Chi tonics and sedatives; tang-kuei and salvia promote Blood circulation and production of new Blood.

TYPICAL VARIATIONS: This is a large **Yuan Dynasty formula,** so it is not often altered. For additional sedative effects and as astringents for nightsweats and nocturnal emission, add dragonbone and oystershell; for weakness of Chi, add astragalus and atractylodes; for Kidney weakness, add cistanche and cuscuta.

1.2 Polygala	Yuanzhi	HT; nourishes Heart,
1.2 Zizyphus	Suanzaoren	sedates Shen
1.2 Biota	Baiziren	
1.2 Asparagus	Tianmendong	HT/LU; nourishes Upper
1.2 Ophiopogon	Maimendong	Warmer Yin
1.2 Salvia	Danshen	HT; vitalizes and
1.2 Tang-kuei	Danggui	nourishes Blood

GINSENG AND ZIZYPHUS FORMULA

1.2 Coptis	Huanglian	HT; purges fire
1.2 Scrophularia	Xuanshen	
1.2 Rehmannia	Shengdihuang	
1.2 Ginseng	Renshen	HT; tonifies Chi,
1.2 Hoelen	Fuling	sedates Heart
1.2 Acorus	Shuichuanpu	HT; opens orifices
1.2 Schizandra	Wuweizi	LU; regulates phlegm
1.2 Platycodon	Jiegeng	

NOTES:

十六味流氣飲

TANG-KUEI SIXTEEN HERB COMBINATION

Shi Liu Wei Liu Qi Yin

LITERAL: Sixteen Ingredients Regulate Chi Special Remedy

THERAPEUTIC PRINCIPLES: disperses stagnant Chi, tonifies Chi and nourishes Blood, enhances immunity functions

INDICATIONS: swellings and lumps, including breast lumps, uterine cysts, skin and lymphatic swelling

PULSE: weak and tight

TONGUE: pale and flaccid

HERBS AND ACTIONS: Lindera, areca seed, magnolia bark, perilla, saussurea, and chih-ko all disperse stagnant Chi; tang-kuei, peony, and cnidium vitalize circulation of Blood and with astragalus, ginseng, and licorice nourish the Blood; cinnamon twig, angelica, and siler promote surface circulation; platycodon resolves masses.

TYPICAL VARIATIONS: This is a large **Ming Dynasty formula** which is usually not modified; for additional blood vitalizing action, add curcuma and corydalis; for soft accumulations, add fritillaria and laminaria; for breast lumps, add cyperus and blue citrus; for skin and lymphatic swelling, add lithospermum; for hard masses, add oyster shell.

3.0 Ginseng	Renshen	SP/LU; tonifies Chi
2.0 Astragalus	Huangqi	
2.0 Licorice	Gancao	
3.0 Tang-kuei	Danggui	LV; nourishes and vitalizes Blood
3.0 Peony	Baishao	
3.0 Cnidium	Chuanxiong	

2.0 Siler	Fangfeng	LU; dispels wind
3.0 Cinnamon	Guizhi	
2.0 Perilla leaf	Zisuye	
2.0 Angelica	Baizhi	
2.0 Lindera	Wuyao	LV/SP; disperses stagnant Chi/Moisture
2.0 Areca seed	Binglang	
2.0 Magnolia bark	Hopo	
2.0 Saussurea	Muxiang	
2.0 Chih-ko	Zhiqiao	
3.0 Platycodon	Jingjie	LU; resolves phlegm

NOTES:

INTRODUCTION TO MA-HUANG

Ma-huang is a powerful herb that disperses Chi from the interior to the surface and opens up the breathing passages. It was the first Chinese herb to be evaluated by Western-trained pharmacologists; it was demonstrated that the main active ingredient is ephedrine which was then shown to have an effect similar to the human hormone norepinephrine (adrenalin). Ephedrine and a second active ingredient, pseudo-ephedrine, are widely used in modern pharmacy for the treatment of lung and sinus congestion.

In general, Ma-huang formulas are utilized for two purposes:

1) To stimulate surface circulation in the treatment of acute disorders (wind invasion) and surface pain. Symptoms include:

feverish feeling or chills
muscle and joint aches, headaches
low energy
floating pulse
lack of perspiration
a congested feeling
itching skin
white tongue coating

2) To enhance respiration in the treatment of asthma, bronchitis, and sinus congestion. Symptoms include:

productive cough
sinus drainage
wheezing
ear infections

Because of the strong dispersing action, persons of weaker constitution usually avoid using Ma-huang formulas, unless

Ma-huang is a minor component in the prescription. In certain combinations, Ma-huang contributes a diuretic effect.

STANDARD MATCHING IN MA-HUANG FORMULAS

APRICOT SEED: added for the treatment of asthmatic breathing. Other anti-asthmatic herbs may also be used, especially for persons of weaker constitution such as ginkgo, morus, perilla fruit, and tussilago.

CINNAMON TWIG: is added for stimulation of surface circulation, for inducing sweating and relieving surface pains. It is often combined with either ginger or peony or both.

GYPSUM: has a fire purging action and is also diuretic; it is added for lung heat syndrome, such as bronchitis, and also for edema.

PUERARIA: is added for surface heat, shoulder/neck tension, and for thirst accompanying an acute febrile disorder.

CAUTIONS ABOUT MA-HUANG FORMULAS

1) Persons who have "reactive asthma," that is, severe asthmatic attacks that arise at very irregular intervals, may experience asthmatic breathing after taking a Ma-huang formula between attacks. To minimize chances of this, the addition of Kidney Yang tonics are recommended; the individual should begin with a low dosage and increase over a period of 3-4 days.

2) Persons with weak constitution, including severe digestive weakness, chronic constipation, or damaged internal organs may find the stimulating effect of Ma-huang to be uncomfortable; the addition of tonics is recommended.

三拗湯

MA-HUANG, LICORICE, AND APRICOT SEED COMBINATION

San Ao Tang

LITERAL: Three Breaks Decoction

THERAPEUTIC PRINCIPLES: open up breathing passages, dispel wind, relieve coughing.

INDICATIONS: asthma, bronchitis, cold, cough.

PULSE: floating, strong

TONGUE: normal

HERBS AND ACTIONS: Ma-huang, apricot seed, and licorice work harmoniously to relieve congestion of the lungs; Ma-huang dispels wind.

TYPICAL VARIATIONS: For Lung heat syndromes, add gypsum (this will produce **Ma-huang and Apricot Seed Combination**); for headache, rhinitis, and general body aches, add atractylodes and cinnamon twig (this will produce **Ma-huang and Atractylodes Combination**); for muscular rheumatism and arthritis, add coix (this will produce **Ma-huang and Coix Combination**); for colds and flus, add cinnamon twig (this will produce **Ma-huang Combination**); for weak individuals with cold or flu, add aconite (this will produce **Ma-huang, Aconite, and Licorice Combination** with apricot seed added); for acute itching of skin accompanying a feverish disorder, add **Cinnamon Combination** (this will produce **Cinnamon and Ma-huang Combination**); for febrile diseases with thirst, add gypsum, cinnamon, ginger, and jujube (this will produce **Major Blue Dragon Combination**).

5.0 Ma-huang	Mahuang	LU; dispels wind, enhances breathing
5.0 Apricot seed	Xingren	LU; arrests cough
5.0 Licorice	Gancao	servant

葛根湯

PUERARIA COMBINATION

Ge Gen Tang

THERAPEUTIC PRINCIPLES: dispel wind, clear surface heat, relax muscles.

INDICATIONS: colds, flus, muscle pain, joint pain.

PULSE: floating, full

TONGUE: slight white coating

HERBS AND ACTIONS: The formula is made from **Cinnamon Combination** by adding pueraria and Ma-huang; it is made from **Ma-huang Combination** by adding pueraria. Pueraria, cinnamon twig, Ma-huang, and ginger dispel wind; peony with cinnamon twig relieves muscle tension; ginger, licorice, and jujube are harmonizers.

TYPICAL VARIATIONS: For severe and recurrent surface tension, add **Minor Bupleurum Combination** (this will produce **Bupleurum and Cinnamon Combination with Ma-huang** and pueraria added); for sinus congestion, add magnolia flower and cnidium (this will produce **Pueraria and Magnolia Combination**); for sinus congestion with inflammation and fever, add cnidium, coix, platycodon, gypsum, and magnolia flower (this will produce **Pueraria Nasal Combination** with rhubarb deleted); for asthmatic breathing, add pinellia, asarum, add schizandra (this will produce **Minor Blue Dragon Combination** with pueraria and jujube added); for severe headache associated with colds, flus, and cough, add cnidium, angelica, cimcifuga, and cyperus (this will produce **Ma-huang and Cimicifuga Combination** with citrus and perilla deleted); for early stage of rheumatoid arthritis, add coix, tang-kuei, peony, and atractylodes (this will produce **Coix Combination** with ginger, jujube, and peuraria added); for back and leg pain, add tu-huo and rehmannia (this will produce **Tu-huo and Pueraria Combination)**

PUERARIA COMBINATION

8.0 Pueraria	Gegen	LU; dispels wind
4.0 Ma-huang	Mahuang	
3.0 Cinnamon	Guizhi	
1.0 Ginger	Shengjiang	
3.0 Peony	Baishao	LV; clears heat, relaxes tension
4.0 Jujube	Dazao	servants
1.0 Licorice	Gancao	

NOTES:

小青龍湯

MINOR BLUE DRAGON COMBINATION

Xiao Qing Long Tang

THERAPEUTIC EFFECTS: dispels wind-chill, decongests lungs and sinuses, relieves allergy reaction.

INDICATIONS: colds, flus, inhalant allergies, asthma, headache, and body aches associated with colds/flus.

PULSE: somewhat slippery; may be floating, slightly weak.

TONGUE: white coating, moist

HERBS AND ACTIONS: Ma-huang decongests lungs and sinuses, and with asarum, ginger, and cinnamon, dispels wind-chill; pinellia, asarum, schizandra, and ginger are expectorants; schizandra strengthens the Lung and normalizes mucus secretions; cinnamon with peony relieves body aches and flushing up of Chi.

TYPICAL VARIATIONS: For flushing up (shoulder/neck tension, headache, sinus congestion), add peuraria; for chill and more severe body aches, add aconite; for chronic asthma, add morus and perilla fruit; for Spleen weakness add codonopsis and jujube; for edema, add hoelen; for severe coughing, add apricot seed; for bronchitis with edema, add hoelen and apricot seed (this will produce **Hoelen and Schizandra Combination** with Ma-huang, cinnamon, and peony added).

3.0 Ma-huang	Mahuang	LU; dispels wind, normalizes breathing
3.0 Asarum	Xixin	
3.0 Cinnamon	Guizhi	
3.0 Schizandra	Wuweizi	
3.0 Ginger	Shengjiang	
3.0 Peony	Baishao	LV; relieves spasms
3.0 Licorice	Gancao	

MINOR BLUE DRAGON COMBINATION

6.0 Pinellia	Banxia	SP/ST; clears Moisture and phlegm

NOTES:

定喘湯

MA-HUANG AND GINKGO COMBINATION

Ting Chuan Tang

LITERAL: Stop Coughing Decoction

THERAPEUTIC PRINCIPLES: disperse stagnant Chi in the chest and Middle Warmer, relieve cough and asthma.

INDICATIONS: persistent cough, difficult breathing.

PULSE: tense, slow

TONGUE: moist

HERBS AND ACTIONS: This formula is made from **Ma-huang, Licorice, and Apricot Seed Combination** by adding additional agents for cough and asthma. Ma-huang decongests the lungs; apricot seed, morus, ginkgo, tussilago, and perilla fruit relieve coughing and wheezing; scute and morus clear deficiency heat and relieve tension in the chest.

TYPICAL VARIATIONS: For copious sputum, add hoelen and citrus (this will produce **Ma-huang and Morus Formula** with ginkgo, tussilago, and scute added); for coughing due to external factors, add peucedanum and perilla leaf.

3.0 Ma-huang	Mahuang	LU; decongests the lungs
1.8 Apricot seed	Xingren	LU; relieves asthma and cough
1.8 Perilla fruit	Zisuzin	
1.8 Morus	Sangbaipi	
4.8 Ginkgo	Baiguo	
3.0 Tussilago	Kuandonghua	
3.0 Pinellia	Banxia	SP/ST; clears Moisture and phlegm

MA-HUANG AND GINKGO COMBINATION

0.6 Scute	Huangqin	LV; purges fire and relieves tension
0.6 Licorice	Gancao	servant

NOTES:

薏苡仁湯

COIX COMBINATION

Yi Yi Ren Tang

THERAPEUTIC PRINCIPLES: activate Chi circulation in the limbs, promote Blood circulation, move Moisture, relieve pain, relieve rheumatism.

INDICATIONS: arthritis, rheumatism, and general body aches, especially in the upper body.

PULSE: strong

TONGUE: white coating

HERBS AND ACTIONS: Ma-huang, atractylodes, cinnamon, and peony relieve surface congestion of Chi and Moisture; tang-kuei and peony promote Blood circulation; coix moves Moisture and relieves rheumatism; licorice is harmonizer.

TYPICAL VARIATIONS: For more severe Moisture accumulation in the limbs, add Tu-huo and hoelen; for shoulder/neck tension, add pueraria; for asthma and edema, add schizandra; for chill, add aconite; for involvement of lower limbs, add anemarrhena, aconite, and siler; for headache, add asarum; for edema with thirst, add hoelen.

4.0 Ma-huang	Mahuang	LU; dispels wind
3.0 Cinnamon	Guizhi	
8.0 Coix	Yiyiren	SP/ST; clears Moisture
4.0 Atractylodes	Baizhu	
4.0 Tang-kuei	Danggui	LV; activates and
3.0 Peony	Baishao	nourishes Blood
2.0 Licorice	Gancao	servant

NOTES:

桂枝芍藥知母湯

CINNAMON AND ANEMARRHENA COMBINATION

Gui Zhi Shao Yao Zhi Mu Tang

THERAPEUTIC PRINCIPLES: dispel wind, warm the Yang

INDICATIONS: rheumatoid arthritis, muscular atrophy of the legs, difficult breathing, paralysis.

PULSE: floating, slow

TONGUE: swollen, white coating

HERBS AND ACTIONS: Cinnamon twig, aconite, and ginger warm the Yang and strengthen the Kidney and Spleen; anemarrhena prevents excessive heating by the warming herbs and helps treat inflammation; siler and ma-huang with cinnamon and ginger dispel wind and relieve surface pain; atractylodes, licorice, and peony tonify Chi and Blood.

TYPICAL ADDITIONS: For Blood deficiency, add tang-kuei, cnidium, rehmannia, astragalus, and hoelen (this will produce **Astragalus and Aconite Formula** with Ma-huang, licorice, ginger, and anemarrhena added); for paralysis and palsy, add stephania, ginseng, scute, cnidium, and apricot seed (this will produce **Ma-huang and Peony Combination** with atractylodes and anemarrhena added); for arthritis of the arms and shoulders, add chiang-huo, asarum, stephania, and hoelen (this will produce **Ma-huang and Chiang-huo Combination** with anemarrhena, peony, and aconite added).

3.0 Ma-huang	Mahuang	LU/BL; dispels wind
3.0 Cinnamon twig	Guizhi	
3.0 Ginger	Ganjiang	
3.0 Siler	Fangfeng	

CINNAMON AND ANEMARRHENA COMBINATION

3.0 Atractylodes	Baizhu	SP/ST; tonifies Chi
1.5 Licorice	Gancao	
3.0 Anemarrhena	Zhimu	LU/KI; clears heat, tonifies Yin
3.0 Peony	Baishao	LU/LV; tonifies Blood, relieves pain
1.0 Aconite	Fuzi	SP/KI; tonifies Yang, relieves pain

NOTES:

INTRODUCTION TO PURGING FIRE AND DISPELLING WIND

Fire purging and wind dispelling therapies are presented together here because the majority of treatments for either fire or wind invasion involve a combination of these herbs. Some formulas presented here are strictly directed at fire purging, but all wind dispelling formulas in this section also contain some fire purging therapy.

Fire purging is a large category of therapy used for treating:

infections	inflammations
red eyes	spontaneous bleeding
short menstrual cycle	fever
dysentery	rashes
hypertension	insomnia
mental distress	headaches
constipation	facial flushing
red tongue	fast, full pulse

These symptoms are similar to those listed for Liver fire (see Bupleurum formulas) and include Liver fire as an underlying cause; however, they may also arise from Heart fire, Stomach fire, Blood heat, and invasion of pathogenic factors that induce heat syndromes (Lung heat). The symptoms are also similar to those of deficiency of Yin (see Yin tonic formulas), except that the fire purging formulas are used when there is little or no Yin deficiency accompanying the heat symptoms.

Wind dispelling formulas treat acute disorders and acute manifestations of internal heat syndromes. They are especially used for:

infections
inflammations
headaches
neuralgia
arthritis
congestion

The range of ingredients in such formulas is quite large, and the range of combining is similarly diverse.

STANDARD MATCHING IN FIRE PURGING AND WIND DISPELLING FORMULAS

COPTIS AND SCUTE: these are utilized in the treatment of internal heat, the excess syndromes of Heart and Liver in particular.

PHELLODENDRON AND GARDENIA: these are used to treat the surface eruption of heat in the form of inflammation, itching, and bleeding; they also treat diarrhea and dysentery.

FORSYTHIA AND LONICERA: these clean toxins and are used when there is an acute infection and also when there are tumors or abscesses.

PUERARIA AND CIMICIFUGA: used for the treatment of skin eruptions, especially rashes, and sinus congestion.

RHUBARB AND MIRABILITUM: these purge the Gallbladder and Colon and clear accumulated heat in the abdomen that is associated with constipation or hard swellings.

GYPSUM AND ANEMARRHENA: used for fire syndrome producing thirst, restlessness, and itching of skin.

CAUTIONS ABOUT FIRE PURGING FORMULAS

1) Most fire purging formulas, if taken over an extended period of time, will cause some gastro-intestinal weakness, including loss of appetite and loose stool. The formulas should be modified by adding digestive tonics, after treatment has proceeded for a period of a few weeks.

2) Wind dispelling herbs may cause uneasiness or nausea in persons of weak constitution (see Ma-huang formulas for a similar caution).

3) The combination of fire purging and wind dispelling also tends to be drying. Therefore, if there is Yin or Blood deficiency or thirst, the formula must be modified by adding the appropriate tonics or moisturizing herbs.

4) Some fire purging formulas rely on the use of the purgative rhubarb root. Some individuals react to rhubarb with intestinal cramping and diarrhea; in such cases, rhubarb must be deleted (lowering the dosage will not resolve the problem).

小承氣湯

MINOR RHUBARB COMBINATION

Xiao Cheng Qi Tang

LITERAL: Minor Chi Resolving Decoction

THERAPEUTIC ACTIONS: purge the Intestines and Gallbladder, purge fire, normalize flow of Chi at the center, dry dampness.

INDICATIONS: constipation, abdominal bloating, acute febrile diseases, hypertension, digestive disturbance with constipation, delirium, dysentery (acute infectious diseases, not for chronic disorder).

PULSE: sinking, full, fast

TONGUE: tends to red; greasy yellow tongue fur

HERBS AND ACTIONS: Rhubarb purges the intestines, and relieves internal heat; chih-shih and magnolia bark are minor purgatives that normalize flow of Chi in the Middle Warmer; all three herbs purge the Gallbladder and help dry dampness.

TYPICAL VARIATIONS: For more severe constipation, add mirabilitum (this produces **Major Rhubarb Combination**); for intestinal dryness and general weakness, add apricot seed, linum, and peony (this produces **Apricot Seed and Linum Formula**); for more severe bloating, add saussurea and areca seed; for delirium, add gambir and hoelen; for Liver tension, add bupleurum, scute, and peony; for dysentery, add saussurea, peony, and phellodendron; for peritonitis, add pinellia and ginger; for acute febrile disease with constipation and bloating, add cinnamon twig, ginger, jujube, and licorice (this will produce **Magnolia Seven Combination**); for uterine carcinoma and pelvic inflammatory disease, add mirabilitum, carthamus, tang-kuei, and licorice (this will produce **Rhubarb and Magnolia Combination**).

MINOR RHUBARB COMBINATION

2.0 Rhubarb	Dahuang	LI; purgative
2.0 Chih-shih	Zhishi	SP/ST; clears accumulation
3.0 Magnolia bark	Houpo	

NOTES:

白虎湯

GYPSUM COMBINATION

Bai Hu Tang

LITERAL: White Tiger Decoction

THERAPEUTIC PRINCIPLES: purges fire.

INDICATIONS: fever, rash, diabetic syndrome, thirst, skin disorders, irritability and mental disturbance.

PULSE: rapid, floating

TONGUE: red

HERBS AND ACTIONS: Gypsum and anemarrhena purge fire; oryza and licorice protect the digestive system from the potential adverse effect of the cold energy herbs.

TYPICAL VARIATIONS: For weakness of Chi, add ginseng (this will produce **Ginseng and Gypsum Combination**); for feverish disorder with phlegm congestion, add platycodon; for skin disorders, add arctium; for acute severe pulmonary disorder with sweating, add ophiopogon, pinellia, ginseng, and bamboo (this will produce **Bamboo Leaves and Gypsum Combination** with anemarrhena added).

15.0 Gypsum	Shigao	LU; purges fire
5.0 Anemarrhena	Zhimu	
8.0 Oryza	Guya	SP/ST; tonifies Chi, harmonizes center
2.0 Licorice	Gancao	

NOTES:

銀翹散

LONICERA AND FORSYTHIA FORMULA

Yin Chiao San

THERAPEUTIC PRINCIPLES: dispel wind-heat in Upper Warmer; relieve inflammation.

INDICATIONS: cold and flu that starts with sore throat, feverish feeling, slight aversion to chills, headache, and thirst (heat-type syndrome); tonsilitis, laryngitis, measles, mumps, skin eruptions, swollen glands.

PULSE: floating and fast

TONGUE: tends to reddish, may have white coating

HERBS AND ACTIONS: Schizonepeta, arctium, and mentha dispel wind-heat in the Upper Warmer; forsythia, lonicera, soja, phragmites, and bamboo leaves relieve internal heat; platycodon, arctium, and forsythia reduce inflammation, and dispel pus.

TYPICAL VARIATIONS: This is a large **Qing Dynasty formula** and is usually not modified; for additional wind-dispelling action, add siler; for headache, add angelica and chrysanthemum; for Yin deficiency, add ophiopogon and anemarrhena; for more severe inflammation, add phellodendron; for lack of vitality, add jujube; for stuffy nose, add magnolia flower and pueraria; for cough, add morus and apricot seed; for severe sore throat, add raw rehmannia and scrophularia; for eruption of measles, add cimicifuga and pueraria.

12.0 Forsythia	Lianqiao	LU; purges fire and cleans toxin
12.0 Lonicera	Jinyinhua	
15.0 Phragmites	Lugen	

LONICERA AND FORSYTHIA FORMULA

9.0 Arctium	Niubangzi	LU; clears surface heat
3.0 Mentha	Bohe	
9.0 Soja	Dandouchi	
6.0 Schizonepeta	Jingjie	
9.0 Bamboo leaves	Zhuye	LU; resolves phlegm
9.0 Platycodon	Jiegeng	

NOTES:

清鼻湯

PUERARIA NASAL COMBINATION

Qing Bi Tang

LITERAL: Clear the Sinuses Decoction

THERAPEUTIC PRINCIPLES: dry dampness in the head, dispel wind, relieve inflammation, dispel pus.

INDICATIONS: sinus congestion, snoring, allergic rhinitis, facial flushing, headaches, earaches, colds/flus with fever, tendency to constipation.

PULSE: full, fast

TONGUE: tends to red, may have yellow coating

HERBS AND ACTIONS: This formula is derived from **Pueraria Combination** (used for treating wind disorders in Yang constitution individuals) by adding herbs specific for nasal congestion and inflammation. Ma-huang, pueraria, and magnolia flower decongest the sinuses; gypsum, coix, rhubarb, peony, and platycodon treat inflammation, heat, and pus in the head; cinammon twig treats flushing up; ginger, jujube, and licorice relieve acute symptoms.

TYPICAL VARIATIONS: For headaches, add chrysanthemum; for lung congestion, increase ma-huang; for dispelling wind (earache, headache, skin eruption, body aches), add siler, angelica, and chiang-huo; for deficient Yin, add anemarrhena, ophiopogon, and lily.

6.0 Pueraria	Gegen	LU; dispel wind
4.0 Magnolia flower	Xinyi	
3.0 Ma-huang	Mahuang	
2.5 Cinnamon	Guizhi	
1.5 Cnidium	Chuanxiong	
1.5 Rhubarb	Dahuang	LI/LV/PC; purge internal fire

PUERARIA NASAL COMBINATION

5.0 Coix	Yiyiren	LU; clear moist heat
2.0 Gypsum	Shigao	LU; purge surface heat
1.5 Peony	Baishao	LV; clear Blood heat
4.5 Platycodon	Jiegeng	LU; clear phlegm
1.5 Ginger	Ganjiang	servants
2.0 Jujube	Dazao	
1.0 Licorice	Gancao	

NOTES:

鈎藤散

GAMBIR FORMULA

Gou Tong San

THERAPEUTIC PRINCIPLES: purges Liver fire, cools the Blood, settles up-rising Chi, strengthens and normalizes function of Spleen and Stomach.

INDICATIONS: hypertensive headaches, insomnia, irritability, nervousness, ringing in the ears, hypertension, neurosis, heart palpitations, menopausal distress, stiff shoulders, eye pain.

PULSE: tense, fast, windy

TONGUE: tends to red

HERBS AND ACTIONS: Gambir relieves Liver and Heart fire, and reduces blood pressure; chrysanthemum and gypsum relieve blood heat and with gambir and siler relieve hypertensive headaches; ophiopogon helps settle rising Chi and with aurantium treats heart palpitation, insomnia, and restlessness; ginseng, licorice, pinellia, and ginger strengthen and normalize the digestive system; hoelen nourishes the Heart and Spleen.

TYPICAL VARIATIONS: For Liver tension, add bupleurum, scute, and peony; for insomnia, add zizyphus; for dry cough, add anemarrhena and ophiopogon; for weak Kidney function, add polyporus and atractylodes; for tinnitus, add polygala and scute; for headache, add pueraria and angelica; for dry skin, add tang-kuei.

5.0 Gypsum	Shigao	LU; purges fire, moistens
3.0 Ophiopogon	Maimendong	
3.0 Gambir	Moutong	LV; purges fire

GAMBIR FORMULA

2.0 Chrysanthemum	Juhua	LU; clears surface heat
2.0 Siler	Fangfeng	
1.0 Ginger	Shengjiang	
2.0 Ginseng	Renshen	SP; tonifies Chi
1.0 Licorice	Gancao	
3.0 Pinellia	Banxia	SP/ST; normalizes functions
3.0 Hoelen	Fuling	
3.0 Aurantium		

NOTES:

黄連解毒湯

COPTIS AND SCUTE COMBINATION

Huang Lian Jie Du Tang

LITERAL: Coptis Clear the Poison Decoction

THERAPEUTIC PRINCIPLES: purges fire, clears toxin, relieves inflammation, stops bleeding, purges damp heat, purges the Gallbladder.

INDICATIONS: spontaneous nosebleed, coughing up blood (hemoptysis), urinary bleeding, hypertension, ringing in the ears, facial flushing, red eyes, insomnia, feverish feeling, itchy skin, boils.

PULSE: sinking, full, fast

TONGUE: red and yellow coating

HERBS AND ACTIONS: Coptis, scute, phellodendron, and gardenia purge fire, eliminate toxins, relieve inflammation, dry dampness, and help stop bleeding.

TYPICAL VARIATIONS: For Yin deficiency, add cooked rehmannia and anemarrhena; for Blood deficiency, add **Tang-kuei Four Combination** (this will produce **Tang-kuei and Gardenia Combination**); for insomnia, add zizyphus; for hot-type diarrhea and for dysentery, add pueraria; for acne rosacea, add carthamus, rehmannia, and peony; for oral inflammation and herpes sores, add mentha and forsythia; for Lower Warmer damp-heat, add tang-kuei, alisma, akebia, and plantago seed; for Upper Warmer damp-heat, add forsythia and mentha; for constipation, add rhubarb (this will produce **Coptis and Rhubarb Combination** with gardenia and phellodendron added); for heartburn, add oyster shell; for dysentery or bloody stool, add pueraria; for boils, ear infection, or conjunctivitis, add siler, mentha, schizonepeta, and forsythia; for extreme thirst, flushing or rashes, and large pulse, add gypsum, ma-huang, soja, and ginger (this will produce **Gypsum, Coptis, and Scute Combination** with jujube and tea deleted).

1.5 Coptis	Huanglian	LV/HT; purges fire,
3.0 Scute	Huangchin	dries dampness
2.0 Gardenia	Zhizi	
1.5 Phellodendron	Huangbai	

NOTES:

當歸拈痛湯

TANG-KUEI AND ANEMARRHENA COMBINATION

Dang Gui Nian Tong Tang

LITERAL: Tang-kuei Get Beyond the Pain Decoction

THERAPEUTIC PRINCIPLES: relieves damp heat, dispels wind heat, tonifies Chi and Blood.

INDICATIONS: pain in the waist, knees, and legs, itching and suppuration of the legs.

PULSE: rapid, floating, soft

TONGUE: swollen, moist

HERBS AND ACTIONS: Capillaris, atractylodes, anemarrhena, scute, polyporus, alisma, and sophora clear damp heat; chiang-huo, siler, cimicifuga, and pueraria dispel wind heat; ginseng, white atractylodes, and licorice tonify Chi and with Tang-kuei nourish the Blood.

TYPICAL VARIATIONS: For more severe edema, add hoelen and cinnamon twig; for reddening and feverish feeling in the joints, add stephania; for anemia, add peony and ho-shou-wu.

1.0 Cimicifuga	Shengma	LU; dispels wind heat
2.0 Pueraria	Gegen	
2.5 Anemarrhena	Zhimu	LU/LV; purges fire
2.5 Scute	Huangqin	
1.0 Sophora	Kushen	
2.5 Capillaris	Yinchen	BL; clears damp heat
2.5 Polyporus	Zhuling	
2.5 Alisma	Zexie	
2.5 Tang-kuei	Danggui	LV; tonifies Blood

2.5 Atractylodes	Baizhu	SP; tonifies Chi
1.0 Licorice	Gancao	

NOTES:

清暑益氣湯

ASTRAGALUS AND ATRACTYLODES COMBINATION

Qing Shu I Qi Tang

LITERAL: Clear Summer Heat and Support the Chi Decoction

THERAPEUTIC PRINCIPLES: tonify Chi, clear heat, disperse stagnant Chi, astringe sweating.

INDICATIONS: feverish disorders with sweating, thirst, cough, and digestive disturbance, degenerative and neurologic diseases.

PULSE: floating, thin, rapid

TONGUE: thin coating, dry

HERBS AND ACTIONS: Ginseng, licorice, astragalus, and atractylodes tonify Chi; tang-kuei nourishes Blood; citrus and blue citrus disperse stagnant Chi; phellodendron, ophiopogon, and alisma purge deficiency fire; pueraria and cimicifuga clear surface heat; schizandra with astragalus astringes sweating; Shen-chu clears stagnant food.

TYPICAL VARIATIONS: This is a large **Yuan Dynasty formula;** it is usually not modified; for dry cough, add anemarrhena; for extreme thirst, add trichosanthes root; for oral ulceration add moutan and cnidium.

2.0 Alisma	Zexie	KI; purges fire
1.0 Phellodendron	Huangbai	
3.0 Ophiopogon	Maimendong	
0.5 Cimicifuga	Shengma	LU; clears surface heat
2.0 Pueraria	Gegen	
3.0 Ginseng	Renshen	SP; tonifies Chi
1.0 Licorice	Gancao	
3.0 Astragalus	Huangqi	
3.0 Atractylodes	Baizhu	

ASTRAGALUS AND ATRACTYLODES COMBINATION

3.0 Citrus	Chenpi	LV; disperses Chi
2.0 Blue Citrus	Qingpi	
3.0 Tang-kuei	Dangqui	LV; tonifies Blood
1.0 Shen-chu	Shenqu	
1.0 Schizandra	Wuweizi	LU; astringes, reduces sweating

NOTES:

龍膽瀉肝湯

GENTIANA COMBINATION

Long Dan Xie Gan Tang

LITERAL: Gentiana Purge the Liver Decoction

THERAPEUTIC PRINCIPLES: purges damp-heat of Lower Warmer, purges fire of Liver, Gallbladder, Heart, and Small Intestine.

INDICATIONS: genital herpes, pelvic inflammatory disease, urinary tract infection with burning sensation, vaginal infection with colored discharge, red eyes, inflammation of tongue, ear infections, headaches.

PULSE: fast, full

TONGUE: reddish tongue, yellow to green coating, especially at sides of tongue

HERBS AND ACTIONS: Gentiana, scute, and gardenia purge fire of the Liver/Gallbladder; akebia and scute purge fire of the Heart and Small Intestine; they all dry dampness; alisma and plantago purge damp-heat of the Lower Warmer; tang-kuei and cooked rehmannia nourish Blood and Yin to counter heat.

TYPICAL VARIATIONS: For Liver tension, add bupleurum and peony; for Small Intestine fire producing Bladder syndromes, add dianthus and polygonum; for constipation, add rhubarb; for Blood stasis in Lower Warmer, add rhubarb, mirabilitum, persica, and leonorus; for burning urination and for kidney gravel, add talc and polyporus; for uterine or urinary bleeding, add gelatin and eclipta; for oral herpes, add forsythia and mentha.

1.0 Gentiana	Longdancao	LV/GB; purges damp heat
5.0 Rehmannia	Dihuang	
3.0 Scute	Huangqin	
1.0 Gardenia	Zhizi	

GENTIANA COMBINATION

5.0 Akebia	Mutong	KI/BL; purges damp heat
3.0 Alisma	Zexie	
9.0 Plantago	Cheqianzi	
5.0 Tang-kuei	Danggui	LV; tonifies Blood
1.0 Licorice	Gancao	servant

NOTES:

葛根紅花湯

PUERARIA AND CARTHAMUS COMBINATION

Ge Gen Hong Hua Tang

THERAPEUTIC PRINCIPLES: clear heat, activate Blood circulation.

INDICATIONS: skin diseases with red patches, vascular inflammation, slow healing acne.

PULSE: rapid, knotty

TONGUE: red

HERBS AND ACTIONS: Carthamus, rhubarb, and pueraria activate circulation of Blood; coptis, gardenia, peony, and raw rehmannia clear heat from the Blood; licorice is harmonizer.

TYPICAL VARIATIONS: For chronic skin disorders, add arctium and sophora; for sudden skin outbreak, add bupleurum and schizonepeta; for more severe blood stasis, add salvia; for abscess, add platycodon and coix.

3.0 Pueraria	Gegen	LU; dispels wind heat
1.5 Carthamus	Honghua	LV; vitalizes Blood
1.0 Rhubarb	Dahuang	
1.5 Coptis	Huanglian	LV; purges fire
1.5 Gardenia	Zhizi	
3.0 Rehmannia	Dihuang	
3.0 Peony	Baishao	
1.0 Licorice	Gancao	servant

NOTES:

清上蠲痛湯

OPHIOPOGON AND ASARUM COMBINATION

Qing Shang Chuan Tong Tang

LITERAL: Cleanse the Top and Relieve Headache Decoction

THERAPEUTIC PRINCIPLES: dispel wind, purge Liver fire.

INDICATIONS: for headache, trigeminal neuralgia, and facial pain

PULSE: floating, may be fast

TONGUE: tends to red; may quiver

HERBS AND ACTIONS: Chiang-huo, Tu-huo, angelica, cnidium, siler, asarum, vitex, and chrysanthemum dispel wind and relieve pain—they are especially effective for the Upper Warmer; ophiopogon calms the up-rushing of Chi; tang-kuei and ginger improve internal circulation; scute, chrysanthemum, and vitex purge Liver fire.

TYPICAL VARIATIONS: This is a large **Ming Dynasty formula;** it is usually not modified; for headaches brought on by the common cold, add schizonepeta and mentha; for migraines, increase the amount of chrysanthemum; for pain focused at the eyes, add cassia seed and tribulus; for hypertension or neurosis, add pinellia and gambir; for thirst, add gypsum.

1.5 Vitex	Manjingzi	LU; dispels wind and wind-heat
1.5 Chrysanthemum	Juhua	
2.5 Siler	Fangfeng	
2.5 Angelica	Baizhi	
1.0 Asarum	Xixin	
2.5 Cnidium	Chuanxiong	
2.5 Chiang-huo	Qianghuo	
1.0 Ginger	Shengjiang	
2.5 Tuhuo	Duhuo	

OPHIOPOGON AND ASARUM COMBINATION

3.0 Scute	Huangqin	LV; purges fire
2.5 Ophiopogon	Maimendong	LU; purges fire, tonifies Yin
2.5 Tang-kuei	Danggui	LV; tonifies Blood
2.0 Atractylodes	Baizhu	SP; tonifies Chi
1.0 Licorice	Gancao	

NOTES:

消風散

TANG-KUEI AND ARCTIUM FORMULA

Xiao Feng San

LITERAL: Eliminate Wind Powder

THERAPEUTIC PRINCIPLES: dispel wind, nourish skin, relieve Blood heat.

INDICATIONS: chronic skin disorders with discharge, itching, or burning (such as eczema); rough and thickened skin; poison oak or ivy rashes.

PULSE: fast, full

TONGUE: red, dry

HERBS AND ACTIONS: Cicada is a specific for chronic skin disease; it is especially good for eczema; tang-kuei, sesame, and arctium also nourish the skin; akebia, gypsum, sophora, and anemarrhena cool Blood heat; siler, schizonepeta, arctium, and cicada dispel wind; rehmannia nourishes Blood and Yin; atractylodes moves Moisture.

TYPICAL VARIATIONS: For upper body skin ailments, add mentha and trichosanthes root; for more severe internal heat, add phellodendron and coptis; for lower body skin ailments, add alisma and capillaris; for Liver tension, add bupleurum and peony; for weaker Blood, add ho-shou-wu, cnidium, and peony; for itching, add tribulus; for joint swelling and inflammation, add clematis, chiang-huo, and alisma; for sore throat and mouth inflammation, add scrophularia and moutan; for acute flare-up of skin conditions, add coix, cimicifuga, and pueraria.

2.0 Arctium	Niubangzi	LU; dispels wind-heat
1.0 Schizonepeta	Jingjie	
1.0 Cicada	Chantui	
2.0 Siler	Fangfeng	

TANG-KUEI AND ARCTIUM FORMULA

1.5 Anemarrhena	Zhimu	LU; purges fire
3.0 Gypsum	Shigao	
3.0 Rehmannia	Dihuang	HT; purges fire, dries dampness, cleans toxin
2.0 Akebia	Mutong	
1.0 Sophora	Kushen	
1.5 Sesame	Huma	LI; moistens dryness
3.0 Tang-kuei	Danggui	
2.0 Atractylodes	Baizhu	SP; tonifies Chi
1.0 Licorice	Gancao	

NOTES:

防風通聖散

SILER AND PLATYCODON COMBINATION

Fang Feng Tong Sheng Tang

LITERAL: Siler Through the Sages Powder

THERAPEUTIC PRINCIPLES: dispel wind, relieve internal heat, purge the Gallbladder and Intestines, increase urinary flow.

INDICATIONS: obesity (in persons with constipation), hypertension, skin disorders, abdominal firmness, stiff and aching shoulders.

PULSE: full, slightly fast

TONGUE: reddish, moist, may have yellow coating

HERBS AND ACTIONS: Rhubarb and mirabilitum relieve constipation; Ma-huang with talc, gypsum, atractylodes, and ginger produces a strong diuretic action; schizonepeta, siler, cnidium, and mentha clear heat and relieve pain and inflammation; gardenia; scute, and forsythia purge fire and dry dampness; Tang-kuei and peony nourish the Blood and relax the Liver; platycodon removes phlegm; licorice is harmonizer.

TYPICAL VARIATIONS: This large formula was written just after Sung Dynasty; it is usually not modified. For obesity, add alisma; for hypertension, add pueraria; for headaches, add chrysanthemum and chiang-huo; for boils, add coptis and phellodendron; for eczema, add arctium; for liver tension, add bupleurum and cyperus; for late onset diabetes, add anemarrhena; for sciatica, add clematis and stephania.

1.5 Rhubarb	Dahuang	LI; purgative
1.5 Mirabilitum	Mangxiao	

SILER AND PLATYCODON COMBINATION

2.0 Scute	Huangqin	LV/HT; purges fire
1.2 Gardenia	Zhizi	
1.2 Forsythia	Lianqiao	
1.2 Schizonepeta	Jingjie	LU; dispels wind
1.2 Siler	Fangfeng	
1.2 Mentha	Pohe	
1.2 Ma-huang	Mahuang	
1.2 Tang-kuei	Danggui	LV; nourishes Blood
1.2 Peony	Baishao	
1.2 Cnidium	Chuanxiong	
3.0 Talc	Huashi	ST; clears heat,
2.0 Gypsum	Shigao	removes Moisture
2.0 Platycodon	Jiegeng	LU; resolves phlegm
2.0 Atractylodes	Baizhu	SP/ST; improves digestion
1.2 Ginger	Ganjiang	
1.2 Licorice	Gancao	

NOTES:

普濟消毒飲

SCUTE AND CIMICIFUGA COMBINATION

Bu Ji Xiao Du Yin

LITERAL TRANSLATION: General Assistance to Eliminate Poison Decoction

THERAPEUTIC PRINCIPLES: purge fire, clear toxins, dissolve phlegm congesting the skin, nerves, and joints, nourish skin, relieve the Liver.

INDICATIONS: sore throat, ear congestion and infection, swollen glands, skin eruptions, cold or flu with fever, restlessness, insomnia, joint pain with inflammation.

PULSE: strong, floating, slippery

TONGUE: tends to red, may have greasy coating.

HERBS AND ACTIONS: Bupleurum and scute relieve the Liver, and with coptis, isatis, forsythia, cimicifuga, and lasiosphaera purge Heart fire, detoxify the Blood, and relieve inflammation; scrophularia, arctium, and platycodon nourish the skin, dispel pus, and relieve inflammation; silkworm, citrus, and platycodon dissolve phlegm congestion, mentha, bupleurum, and cimicifuga clear surface heat; licorice is harmonizer.

TYPICAL VARIATIONS: This is a large **Qing Dynasty formula** that is usually not modified; for thick sputum, add trichosanthes seed and bamboo leaves; for constipation add gardenia; for inflammation of the mouth, add gypsum and raw rehmannia; for severe thirst, add alisma and gypsum.

6.0 Bupleurum	Chaihu	LV/GB; disperses Chi, purges fire
9.0 Scute	Huangqin	
6.0 Coptis	Huanglian	

SCUTE AND CIMICIFUGA COMBINATION

12.0 Forsythia	Lianqiao	LV/HT/LU; purges fire, cleans toxin
9.0 Scrophularia	Xuanshen	
12.0 Isatis	Daqinye	
3.0 Lasiosphera	Mabo	
4.5 Mentha	Bohe	LU; clears surface heat
9.0 Arctium	Nuzhenzi	
2.4 Cimicifuga	Shengma	
3.0 Platycodon	Jiegeng	LU; clears phlegm
6.0 Silkworm		
3.0 Citrus	Chenpi	SP; servants
3.0 Licorice	Gancao	

NOTES:

洗肝明目湯

GARDENIA AND VITEX COMBINATION

Xie Gan Ming Mu Tang

LITERAL: Clear the Liver to Brighten the Eyes Decoction

THERAPEUTIC PRINCIPLES: purge Liver fire, dispel wind, nourish the eyes.

INDICATIONS: eye diseases marked by inflammation or clouding.

PULSE: fast, full

TONGUE: red

HERBS AND ACTIONS: The formula is made from **Tang-kuei Four Combination** (which nourishes the Blood and benefits the eyes) and **Coptis and Scute Combination** (with phellodendron replaced by forsythia) to purge fire of the Liver and Heart; wind dispelling herbs such as Chiang-huo, mentha, and siler are added, as well as herbs known to benefit the eyes specifically: chyrsanthemum, tribulus, vitex, and cassia seed. The formula also contains platycodon, gypsum, and licorice to treat acute symptoms.

TYPICAL VARIATIONS: This very large **Ming Dynasty formula** is usually not modified; for Yin deficiency of Liver, add lycium fruit.

1.0 Schizonepeta	Jingjie	LU; dispels wind
1.0 Chrysanthemum		
1.0 Tribulus		
1.5 Siler		
1.0 Mentha		
1.0 Vitex		
1.0 Chiang-huo		

GARDENIA AND VITEX COMBINATION

1.5 Tang-kuei	Danggui	LV; tonifies Blood
1.5 Peony		
1.5 Cnidium		
1.5 Rehmannia		
1.5 Forsythia	Lianqiao	LV/HT; purges fire
1.5 Coptis		
1.5 Scute		
1.5 Gardenia		
3.0 Gypsum		
1.0 Platycodon	Jiegeng	SP; servants
1.0 Licorice		

NOTES:

紫根牡蠣湯

LITHOSPERMUM AND OYSTER SHELL COMBINATION

Zi Gen Mu Li Tang

THERAPEUTIC PRINCIPLES: clean toxin, vitalize Blood, nourish Blood.

INDICATIONS: skin and lymphatic system swellings and tumors.

PULSE: rapid, pecking

TONGUE: pale with red spots

HERBS AND ACTIONS: Lonicera, lithospermum, and cimicifuga clear heat and toxins; tang-kuei, peony, and cnidium with astragalus nourish the Blood and with rhubarb vitalize Blood circulation; oyster shell helps resolve firm masses; licorice is harmonizer.

TYPICAL VARIATIONS: For additional detoxification and antitumor activity, add oldenlandia, houttuynia, and coix; for hard mass in the lymphatic system, add sargassum and laminaria; for more severe blood stasis, add salvia and myrrh; for leukorrhea, add smilax, citrus, akebia, and hoelen (this will produce **Tang-kuei Eight Herb Combination** with peony, oyster shell, cimicifuga, licorice, and lithospermum added).

3.0 Lithospermum	Zicao	HT; purges fire,
1.5 Lonicera	Jinyinhua	cleans toxins
1.5 Cimicifuga	Shengma	LU; cleans toxin
5.0 Tang-kuei	Danggui	LV; vitalizes and
3.0 Peony	Shaoyao	tonifies Blood
3.0 Cnidium	Chuanxiong	
4.0 Oyster shell	Muli	LV/GB; purges fire, softens mass

LITHOSPERMUM AND OYSTER SHELL COMBINATION

1.5 Rhubarb	Dahuang	LV; purges fire, vitalizes Blood
2.0 Astragalus	Huangqi	SP; tonifies Chi
1.0 Licorice	Gancao	

NOTES:

辛夷清肺湯

MAGNOLIA AND GYPSUM COMBINATION

Xin Yi Qing Re Tang

LITERAL: Magnolia Flower Clean the Lungs Decoction

THERAPEUTIC PRINCIPLES: purge fire, dispel wind, tonify Yin.

INDICATIONS: nasal congestion, sinus inflammation.

PULSE: rapid, floating

TONGUE: reddish, dry

HERBS AND ACTIONS: Magnolia flower and cimicifuga help relieve sinus congestion; eriobotrya lowers uprising Chi; lily and ophiopogon clear heat and nourish Yin of the Lungs; scute, gardenia, anemarrhena, and gypsum purge fire.

TYPICAL VARIATIONS: For recalcitrant sinus congestion, add xanthium fruit; for accompanying sore throat, add raw rehmannia and moutan; for accompanying coughing, add tussilago and morus bark.

2.0 Magnolia flower	Xinyi	LU; dispels wind
1.0 Cimicifuga	Shengma	
5.0 Gypsum	Shigao	LU; purges fire
3.0 Anemarrhena	Zhimu	
3.0 Gardenia	Zhizi	
1.0 Scute	Huangqin	
3.0 Lily	Baihe	LU; tonifies Yin
5.0 Ophiopogon	Maimendong	
2.0 Eriobotrya	Pipaye	LU; relieves uprushing Chi

十味敗毒湯

BUPLEURUM AND SCHIZONEPETA

Shi Wei Bai Du Tang

LITERAL: Ten Ingredients Remove Toxin Decoction

THERAPEUTIC PRINCIPLES: dispel wind, detoxify Blood.

INDICATIONS: acne and other recurrent skin inflammations.

PULSE: tense

TONGUE: somewhat red

HERBS AND ACTIONS: Bupleurum, schizonepeta, tu-huo, cnidium, ginger, and siler dispel wind; schizonepeta, cnidium, and cherry bark (can be replaced by forsythia if not available) stimulate detoxification by the Liver; platycodon dispels pus; hoelen clears excess moisture; ginger and licorice are servants.

TYPICAL VARIATIONS: For Blood deficiency, add **Tang-kuei Four Combination;** for more severe skin eruptions, add chih-ko, chiang-huo, mentha, forsythia, and lonicera (this will produce Schizonepeta and Siler Combination with cherry bark replacing peucedanum); for skin itching, add tribulus, xanthium, and mentha; for rashes, add gypsum and anemarrhena; for purplish skin eruptions, add salvia and carthamus.

3.0 Bupleurum	Chaihu	LV; detoxifies, dispels wind
1.0 Schizonepeta	Jingjie	
3.0 Cnidium	Chuangxiong	
3.0 Cherry bark	Yingpi	
2.0 Tu-huo	Tuhuo	BL; removes surface Moisture
2.0 Hoelen	Fuling	
3.0 Platycodon	Jiegeng	LU; clears phlegm and pus
1.0 Ginger	Ganjiang	servants
1.0 Licorice	Gancao	

INTRODUCTION TO YIN TONICS

Yin tonics are nourishing, moisturizing, calming herbs used for the treatment of symptoms such as:

thirst	dryness
agitation	insomnia
chronic inflammation	thready pulse
red tongue	thready, fast pulse
constipation	back ache
dry cough	ringing in the ears

Although there are many possible combinations of Yin tonic herbs, most practitioners rely upon the use of Rehmannia Six Formula and its variations. Rehmannia is the primary Yin tonic herb, and is especially suitable for treating deficiency affecting the Kidney and Liver, that is, with symptoms involving the lower body and the eyes and ears.

However, an equally important Yin tonic herb is ophiopogon, which is more suited for Yin deficiency affecting the Lungs, Stomach, and Heart. It is used for symptoms of excessive sweating, dry cough, insomnia, and stomach distress.

STANDARD MATCHING WITH REHMANNIA

ALISMA: to reduce the greasy quality of rehmannia and to direct the herb to treatment of deficiency fire of the Kidney.

CORNUS: to treat impotence, back ache, and weakness of the lower body in general.

DENDROBIUM: to treat damaged Yin due to severe feverish disorder

LYCIUM FRUIT: to nourish the Kidney Essence, usually in combination with eucommia and disoscorea

ANEMARRHENA AND PHELLODENDRON: to clear deficiency fire

MOUTAN: to clear heat from the Blood

STANDARD MATCHING WITH OPHIOPOGON

ASPARAGUS: for cough with thick sputum

SCHIZANDRA: for productive cough

TRICHOSANTHES ROOT: for thirst related to feverish disorders

ANEMARRHENA AND PHELLODENDRON: to clear deficiency fire

SCROPHULARIA: for swollen glands, thirst, and sore throat.

GINSENG: for diabetes, digestive disorders, and dry cough.

CAUTIONS ABOUT USING YIN TONIC FORMULAS

1) Because of their moisturizing quality, Yin tonics may exacerbate congestion of moisture and phlegm. For persons with this type of problem, the inclusion of fragrant Moisture and

Chi resolving herbs, such as cardamon, saussurea, and magnolia bark, may be helpful.

2) Many times, the condition of Yin deficiency of the Kidney is also accompanied by some Yang deficiency. If no Yang tonics are included in the formula, it is possible that the person will respond by feeling cold and lethargic. Warm and spicy Yang tonics will help avoid this problem. In the contrary case, where a formula with Yang tonics is given and causes the individual to feel hot and dry, this means that the Yin deficiency is the more pronounced problem and herbs to treat deficiency fire should be included in the formula, with less reliance on the Yang tonics.

滋陰降火湯

PHELLODENDRON COMBINATION

Su Yin Jiang Huo Tang

LITERAL: Moisten the Yin, Reduce the Fire Decoction

THERAPEUTIC PRINCIPLES: nourish Yin and Blood, purge fire.

INDICATIONS: Lung-heat diseases, facial flushing, feverish feeling, diabetes, thirst, nightsweats, constipation.

PULSE: thin, fast, weak

TONGUE: dry, cracked

HERBS AND ACTIONS: Asparagus, ophiopogon, anemarrhena, and rehmannia are sweet, moist tonics to nourish the Yin; tang-kuei and peony nourish the Blood; phellodendron purges deficiency fire; citrus and atractylodes dispel stagnant Chi; licorice is harmonizer.

TYPICAL VARIATIONS: For difficult expectoration add trichosanthes seed and bamboo leaves; for drier cough, add lily and eriobotrya; for mouth sores, add scrophularia and moutan; for constipation, add cannabis seed and persica; for nightsweats, add astragalus; for diabetes, add dioscorea and cornus; for pruritis, add tribulus; for reduced sexual energy, add lycium fruit and lotus seed.

2.5 Rehmannia	Dihuang	KI/LU; nourishes Yin, purges fire
2.5 Ophiopogon	Maimendong	
2.5 Asparagus	Tiandong	
1.5 Anemarrhena	Zhimu	KI; purges fire
1.5 Phellodendron	Huangbai	
2.5 Tang-kuei	Danggui	LV; nourishes and activates Blood
2.5 Peony	Baishao	

PHELLODENDRON COMBINATION

2.5 Citrus	Chenpi	SP; disperses Chi
3.0 Atractylodes	Baizhu	SP/ST; tonifies Chi
1.5 Licorice	Gancao	

NOTES:

六味地黄丸

REHMANNIA SIX FORMULA

Liu Wei Di Huang Wan

THERAPEUTIC ACTIONS: nourish the Yin, strengthen Kidney and Spleen, astringe and consolidate Chi.

INDICATIONS: thirst, dry skin, constipation with dryness, low back ache, weakness of the knees and lower limbs, late afternoon fatigue and feverish feeling, heat of the palms and soles, nightsweats, general weakness.

TONGUE: shrunken, red, dry

PULSE: thin and weak, fast

HERBS AND ACTIONS: Rehmannia is a heavy, moist Yin tonic, especially suitable for nourishing Kidney Yin, also nourishing the Blood; alisma purges Kidney deficiency fire, and with dioscorea and hoelen strengthens the Spleen; cornus astringes and consolidates Chi and nourishes Liver Yin; moutan purges deficiency fire.

TYPICAL ADDITIONS: For eye swelling, dryness, or blurring of vision, add lycium fruit and chrysanthemum (this produces **Lycium, Chrysanthemum, and Rehmannia Formula);** for asthma and weak immune system, add schizandra (this produces **Rehmannia and Schizandra Formula);** for frequent urination and for diabetes, add cinnamon bark and aconite (this produces **Rehmannia Eight Formula);** for prostatitis and kidney stones, add achyranthes, plantago, cinnamon bark, and aconite (this will produce **Achyranthes and Plantago Formula);** for severe deficiency fire, add anemarrhena and phellodendron (this produces **Anemarrhena, Phellodendron, and Rehmannia Formula);** for severe nightsweats add cuscuta and lotus stamen; for Liver tension and anemia, add **Bupleurum and Peony Formula.**

REHMANNIA SIX FORMULA

6.0 Rehmannia 3.0 Alisma	Dihuang Zexie	KI; nourishes Yin, purges fire
3.0 Cornus 3.0 Moutan	Shanzhuyu Mudanpi	LV; nourishes Yin, cools Blood
3.0 Dioscorea 3.0 Hoelen	Shanyao Fuling	KI/SP; tonifies Chi, clears Moisture

NOTES:

還少丹

LYCIUM FORMULA

Huan Shao Dan

LITERAL: Returning of Youth Elixir

THERAPEUTIC PRINCIPLES: supplement Kidney Yang, strengthen the five organ systems.

INDICATIONS: weak knees, low back ache, impotence, general weakness, night sweats, diabetes, chill, developmental disorders, constipation.

PULSE: weak, slow

TONGUE: pale, moist

HERBS AND ACTIONS: Fennel, cornus, dioscorea, cistanche, lycium, eucommia, achyranthes, morinda, rehmannia, and broussonetia supplement Kidney and Liver; hoelen, jujube, and discorea strengthen the Spleen; acorus, polygala, and hoelen strengthen Kidney and Heart; schizandra strengthens Kidney and Lung.

TYPICAL VARIATIONS: To nourish Blood, add ho-shou-wu; to nourish the Yin, add ligustrum; for menstrual bleeding, add epimedium; for weaker digestion, add codonopsis and licorice; for night sweats, add oyster shell; for insomnia, add zizyphus; for seminal emission, add cuscuta; for low back ache, add eucommia.

1.2 Rehmannia	Dihuang	KI; nourishes Yin
1.2 Cornus	Shanzhuyu	
1.2 Lycium	Gouqizi	
1.2 Eucommia	Duzhong	KI; tonifies Yang
1.2 Morinda	Bajitan	
1.2 Cistanche	Roucongrong	

LYCIUM FORMULA

1.2 Fennel	Xiaohuexiang	SP; tonifies Chi
1.2 Dioscorea	Shanyao	
4.0 Jujube	Dazao	
1.2 Hoelen	Fuling	KI; clears Moisture
1.2 Broussonetia	Qushi	
1.2 Acorus	Shichangpu	HT; benefits wisdom
1.2 Polygala	Yuanzhi	
1.2 Achyranthes	Niuxi	LV; strengthens lower body
1.2 Schizandra	Wuweizi	KI; astringes Essence

NOTES:

百合固金湯

LILY COMBINATION

Bai Ho Gu Jin Tang

LITERAL: Lily Strengthen the Metal Element Decoction

THERAPEUTIC PRINCIPLES: tonify Lung Yin, nourish Blood, dissolve heated phlegm.

INDICATIONS: dry cough, hoarseness, feverish feeling, expectorating blood, restlessness, vivid dreaming, insomnia.

PULSE: rapid, very thin

TONGUE: red, shrunken, little or no coating

HERBS AND ACTIONS: Lily, fritillaria, ophiopogon, scrophularia, and rehmannia moisten the Lung and purge fire; tang-kuei and peony nourish Blood; platycodon resolves phlegm; licorice is harmonizer.

TYPICAL VARIATIONS: For chronic wheezing, add scute and morus; for swollen glands, add trichosanthes root and bamboo; for weakness of Chi, add codonopsis and atractylodes.

4.0 Lily	Baihe	LU/HT; nourishes Yin,
4.0 Rehmannia	Dihuang	purges fire
6.0 Ophiopogon	Maimendong	
3.0 Scrophularia	Xuanshen	
4.0 Tang-kuei	Danggui	LV; nourishes Blood
3.0 Peony	Baishao	
2.0 Platycodon	Jiegeng	LU; disperses phlegm
3.0 Fritillaria	Beimu	
0.5 Licorice	Gancao	servant

NOTES:

清肺湯

PLATYCODON AND FRITILLARIA COMBINATION

Qing Fei Tang

LITERAL: Clean the Lungs Decoction

THERAPEUTIC PRINCIPLES: tonify Lung Chi, nourish Lung Yin, disperse heated phlegm, relieve deficiency fire.

INDICATIONS: severe productive cough with thick mucus, thirst, fever.

PULSE: fast, thin, congested

TONGUE: dry, reddish

HERBS AND ACTIONS: Schizandra, platycodon, and morus nourish Lung Chi; ophiopogon, fritillaria, and asparagus nourish Lung Yin; apricot seed, bamboo, citrus, and hoelen are expectorants; scute and gardenia purge Liver fire; tang-kuei nourishes blood; ginger, jujube, and licorice aid the treatment of acute symptoms.

TYPICAL VARIATIONS: This is a large Ming Dynasty formula and is usually not modified; for Liver tension, add bupleurum; for sore throat, add forsythia; if the mucus is colored, add trichosanthes seed.

3.0 Ophiopogon	Maimendong	LU; nourishes Yin,
2.0 Asparagus	Tianmendong	purges fire
2.0 Bamboo	Zhuru	LU; resolves heated
2.0 Fritillaria	Beimu	phlegm
2.0 Platycodon	Jiegeng	
2.0 Scute	Huangqin	LU; purges fire
2.0 Gardenia	Zhizi	

PLATYCODON AND FRITILLARIA COMBINATION

2.0 Morus	Sangbaipi	LU; relieves cough
2.0 Apricot seed	Xingren	
3.0 Tang-kuei	Danggui	LV; nourishes Blood
2.0 Citrus	Chenpi	SP; clears Moisture
3.0 Hoelen	Fuling	
0.5 Schizandra	Wuweizi	LU; regulates sputum
0.5 Ginger	Ganjiang	servants
3.0 Jujube	Dazao	
1.0 Licorice	Gancao	

NOTES:

補陰湯

TANG-KUEI AND REHMANNIA COMBINATION

Bu Yin Tang

LITERAL: Supplement the Yin Decoction

THERAPEUTIC PRINCIPLES: nourish the Yin, supplement Kidney Yang; purge deficiency fire.

INDICATIONS: low back ache, weak knees, sciatica, dry skin, abdominal bleeding, feverish feeling, impotence, general weakness.

PULSE: weak, thin, rapid

TONGUE: dry

HERBS AND ACTIONS: Ginseng, psoralea, eucommia, achyranthes, and fennel support the upward flow of Chi, strengthening the knees, waist, and lower back; they help overcome impotence and improve vitality; anemarrhena and rehmannia nourish the Yin; tang-kuei and peony nourish the Blood to support the Yin; citrus dispels stagnant chi and hoelen moves stagnant moisture; licorice is harmonizer.

TYPICAL VARIATIONS: This is a large **Ming Dynasty formula;** it is usually not modified. For pain in the lower limbs, add chin-chiu; for nephritis, add stephania and astragalus; for severe deficiency fire, increase the phellodendron and anemarrhena; for anemia, add ho-shou-wu and lycium; for uterine bleeding, add gelatin and artemesia; for constipation, add cistanches; for prostate inflammation, add alisma and talc; for diabetes, add cornus, alisma, and dioscorea; for reduced sexual energy, increase the amount of fennel and add lycium fruit; for abdominal bloating, add saussurea.

TANG-KUEI AND REHMANNIA COMBINATION

2.0 Rehmannia	Dihuang	KI; nourishes Yin, purges fire
1.0 Anemarrhena	Zhimu	
1.0 Phellodendron	Huangbai	
2.0 Eucommia	Duzhong	KI; tonifies Yang
2.0 Psoralea	Buguzhi	
3.0 Tang-kuei	Danggui	LV; nourishes and activates Blood
2.0 Peony	Baishao	
2.0 Achyranthes	Niuxi	
2.0 Ginseng	Renshen	SP; tonifies Chi
1.0 Licorice	Gancao	
1.0 Fennel	Xiaohuexiang	SP/ST; normalizes functions
2.0 Citrus	Chenpi	
3.0 Hoelen	Fuling	

NOTES:

清熱補血湯

CNIDIUM AND MOUTAN COMBINATION

Qing Re Bu Xue Tang

LITERAL: Decoction to Clear Heat and Tonify Blood

THERAPEUTIC PRINCIPLES: nourish Blood and Yin, relieve deficiency fire.

INDICATIONS: feverish feeling, inflammation of the tongue, mouth sores, sore throat, chronic dry cough, dry skin, constipation, anemia, general weakness, night sweats, diabetes, immune system disorders.

PULSE: fast, thin or hollow

TONGUE: reddish, dry

HERBS AND ACTIONS: This formula is comprised of the Blood tonic Tang-kuei Four Combination with the Yin tonic, fire purging anemarrhena, ophiopogon, and scrophularia added; phellodendron, coptis, bupleurum, and moutan purge fire and clear Blood heat; schizandra is a tonic and astringent.

TYPICAL VARIATIONS: This is a large **Ming Dynasty formula** and is usually not modified; for swollen glands, add platycodon and bamboo; for more severe inflammation, add forsythia and gardenia; for insomnia and mental distress, add longan and zizyphus; for chronic dry cough, add trichosanthes seed and scute; for dry constipation, add linum and persica; for loss of hearing or tinnitus, add scute, angelica, and cyperus; for abdominal swelling, add citrus; for thirst, add gypsum.

3.0 Ophiopogon	Maimendong	LU; nourishes Yin,
1.5 Schizandra	Wuweizi	regulates fluid

CNIDIUM AND MOUTAN COMBINATION

1.5 Scrophularia	Xuanshen	KI; purges deficiency fire
1.5 Anemarrhena	Zhimu	
1.5 Phellodendron	Huangbai	
1.5 Moutan	Mudanpi	
3.0 Tang-kuei	Danggui	LV; nourishes Blood
3.0 Peony	Baishao	
3.0 Cnidium	Chuanxiong	
3.0 Rehmannia	Dihuang	
1.5 Bupleurum	Chaihu	LV; clears surface heat

NOTES:

麥門冬湯

OPHIOPOGON COMBINATION

Mai Men Dong Tang

THERAPEUTIC PRINCIPLES: nourish Lung and Stomach Yin, strengthen Spleen.

INDICATIONS: dry cough, facial flushing, thirst, profuse sticky sputum, hoarseness, dry skin, diabetes, and immune system disorders.

PULSE: thin, weak

TONGUE: dry

HERBS AND ACTIONS: Ophiopogon nourishes the Yin, especially Lung Yin, and helps settle uprushing Chi; ginseng and oryza strengthen the Spleen and aid normal production of mucus; pinellia is an expectorant; jujube and licorice are Chi tonics.

TYPICAL VARIATIONS: For drier coughs, add lily and asparagus; for productive cough with thick mucus, add fritillaria, morus, and bamboo; for accompanying digestive disorder, add ginger and citrus; for Lung heat and Blood heat, add gypsum and anemarrhena; for asthma, add perilla fruit and schizandra; for severe hacking cough, add eriobotrya and apricot seed; for hypertension and atherosclerosis, add gambir, gypsum, and chyrsanthemum; for emphysema, add bamboo leaves and gypsum (this will produce Bamboo Leaves and Gypsum Combination); for constipation, add linum and cooked rehmannia.

10.0 Ophiopogon	Maimendong	LU; nourishes Yin,
2.0 Ginseng	Renshen	SP; tonifies Chi
2.0 Licorice	Gancao	
3.0 Jujube	Dazao	
5.0 Pinellia	Banxia	SP/ST; normalizes
5.0 Oryza	Guya	function

INTRODUCTION TO BLOOD ACTIVATING HERBS

Tang-kuei is the primary herb involved in treating blood disorders; it tonifies the blood, activates blood circulation, and aids in detoxification. However, there are other herbs which are used for "cracking" static blood, notably moutan, persica, myrrh, mastic, and carthamus. These have a stronger action on tumors, abscesses, menstrual disorders, and degenerative arthritis. This section features these potent blood activating prescriptions, plus the basic Tang-kuei Four Combination for tonifying and activating blood which may be used for milder conditions where deficiency is predominant.

Blood activating formulas are indicated with the following symptoms:

sharp pains
abscesses
female infertility
knotty pulse
tumors
severe inflammation
purple spots on the tongue
traumatic injuries

STANDARD MATCHING OF HERBS IN BLOOD ACTIVATING FORMULAS

PERSICA AND CARTHAMUS: these are combined for cracking static blood, and especially for pain in the lower abdomen.

MYRRH AND MASTIC: these are resins that are combined for vitalizing blood especially in the skin, arteries, and traumatized tissues; they aid regeneration of new tissues.

CINNAMON TWIG AND PEONY: are combined to relax the blood vessels, especially good for muscular disorders.

TANG-KUEI AND CNIDIUM: are combined for blood stasis affecting the Liver meridian, such as breast and groin swellings.

CAUTIONS ABOUT BLOOD ACTIVATING FORMULAS

1) Blood activation may cause nausea or gastro-intestinal distress in some people; in such cases the herbs should be taken after meals and along with carminative herbs.

2) If there is blood heat, blood activating herbs may cause spontaneous bleeding; in cases where blood heat is a symptom, the appropriate fire purging herbs should be added; if bleeding is already a problem, hemostatics must be added.

騰龍湯

MOUTAN AND PERSICA COMBINATION

Deng Long Tang

LITERAL: Tame the Dragon Decoction

THERAPEUTIC PRINCIPLES: activate Blood circulation, relieve inflammation, clear dampness.

INDICATIONS: severe inflammation and swelling of lower abdomen.

PULSE: rapid, full, deep

TONGUE: may have purplish areas, coated yellow in back

HERBS AND ACTIONS: This formula is made from **Rhubarb and Moutan Combination** by adding coix, atractylodes, and licorice; it is also made from **Benincassa Combination** by adding atractylodes, rhubarb, and mirabilitum. Moutan, persica, rhubarb, and mirabilitum activate Blood circulation and break up the hard mass; coix, benincassa, and atractylodes remove accumulated moisture and relieve inflammation; licorice is harmonizer.

TYPICAL VARIATIONS: For more severe toxic syndrome, add forsythia and lonicera; for severe pain, add zedoria and cyperus; for edema, add hoelen and alisma; for facial flushing, add cinnamon and pueraria.

4.0 Moutan	Mudanpi	LV; vitalizes Blood
4.0 Persica	Taoren	
4.0 Atractylodes	Baizhu	SP/ST; moves Moisture
8.0 Coix	Yiyiren	
5.0 Benincasa	Dongguazi	
1.5 Rhubarb	Dahuang	LI; purges;
5.0 Mirabilitum	Mangxiao	resolves mass

四物湯

TANG-KUEI FOUR COMBINATION

Si Wu Tang

LITERAL: Decoction of Four Substances

THERAPEUTIC PRINCIPLES: nourish Blood, activate Blood circulation; relieve pain; moisturize skin and colon.

INDICATIONS: anemia, menstrual irregularity, uterine bleeding; dry skin, constipation.

PULSE: hollow, or sinking, weak

TONGUE: pale

HERBS AND ACTIONS: Tang-kuei, cnidium, peony, and rehmannia nourish Blood; tang-kuei, cnidium, and peony activate Blood circulation and relieve pain; tang-kuei and rehmannia moisturize the colon.

TYPICAL VARIATIONS: With weak Spleen Chi, add **Four Major Herbs Combination** (this will produce **Tang-kuei and Ginseng Eight Combination**); with more severe blood stasis in strong constitution individual, add Cinnamon and Hoelen Combination; for persistent leukorrhea, uterine bleeding, or other vaginal discharge, add Coptis and Scute Combination (this will produce **Tang-kuei and Gardenia Combination**); for persistent uterine bleeding, add artemesia, gelatin, and licorice (this will produce **Tang-kuei and Gelatin Combination**); for threatened abortion, add white atractylodes and scute (this will form **Tang-kuei Formula** with rehmannia added); for infertility, habitual abortion, and other disorders of pregnancy, add white atractylodes, hoelen, and alisma (this will form **Tang-kuei and Peony Combination** with rehmannia added); for anemia and heart palpitation, add cinnamon bark, hoelen, atractylodes, and licorice (this will produce **Tang-kuei and Atractylodes Combination**).

TANG-KUEI FOUR COMBINATION

4.0 Tang-kuei	Danggui	LV; nourishes and
4.0 Cnidium	Chuanxiong	vitalizes Blood
4.0 Peony	Baishao	
4.0 Rehmannia	Dihuang	

NOTES:

桂枝茯苓丸

CINNAMON AND HOELEN COMBINATION

Gui Zhi Fu Ling Wan

THERAPEUTIC ACTIONS: opens the vessels, activates Blood circulation, dispels Blood stasis.

INDICATIONS: Blood stasis in Lower Warmer, abdominal pain, headache, sinus congestion, constipation, excess weight in pelvis, low back ache, menstrual irregularity, nervousness, fatigue, skin eruptions, uterine tumors, scanty menstrual flow.

PULSE: sinking, tense, congested

TONGUE: may be pale with purplish spots; white coating

HERBS AND ACTIONS: Cinnamon twig opens the vessels; persica, moutan, and peony activate Blood circulation; cinnamon and hoelen relieve accumulation of Moisture.

TYPICAL VARIATIONS: For anemia, add tang-kuei and cnidium; for menstrual pain, add cnidium, zedoria, and corydalis; for edema and scanty urine, add alisma; for Liver tension, add bupleurum and cyperus; for Chi tonification, add codonopsis; for Blood stasis following miscarriage or abortion, add carthamus; for uterine tumor, add bupleurum, chih-ko, coix, and licorice; for menstrual pain, add cnidium, tang-kuei, carthamus, corydalis, and achyranthes (this will produce **Cinnamon and Persica Combination** with hoelen added); for internal chill, add ginger (this will produce **Ginger, Cinnamon, and Hoelen Combination**).

4.0 Cinnamon	Guizhi	LV; relaxes the vessels
4.0 Peony	Baishao	

CINNAMON AND HOELEN COMBINATION

4.0 Moutan	Mudanpi	LV; activates Blood circulation
4.0 Persica	Taoren	
4.0 Hoelen	Fuling	KI; clears Moisture

NOTES:

疏經活血湯

CLEMATIS AND STEPHANIA COMBINATION

Shu Jing Huo Xie Tang

LITERAL: Decoction for Clearing the Vessels and Activating Blood

THERAPEUTIC PRINCIPLES: dispel Blood stasis, activate Blood circulation, nourish the Blood, relieve pain, dispel wind, move Moisture, strengthen Spleen.

INDICATIONS: arthritis, neuralgia, sciatica, gout, lumbago, knee pain; especially pains in the lower body.

PULSE: sinking, congested

TONGUE: may have purple spots; no tongue fur

HERBS AND ACTIONS: The formula is made from **Tang-kuei Four Combination** with the addition of wind-dispelling and blood activating herbs; peony, cnidium, persica, achyranthes, and tang-kuei dispel Blood stasis, activate Blood circulation, and nourish Blood; chiang-huo, angelica, clematis, and siler open the vessels, dispel wind, and relieve pain; chin-chiu and achyranthes improve circulation in the lower part of the body; hoelen and atractylodes move Moisture and with licorice, citrus and ginger, strengthen the Spleen; licorice is harmonizer.

TYPICAL VARIATIONS: This is a large **Ming Dynasty formula;** it is usually not modified; for weakness in lower body, add eucommia; for more severe Blood stasis, add carthamus and red peony; for abdominal pain, add corydalis and zedorea; for constipation, add gardenia; for more severe dampness at the surface, add tu-huo; for phlegm congestion, add arisaema and phellodendron.

2.0 Persica	Taoren	LV; vitalizes Blood
1.5 Achyranthes	Niuxi	

CLEMATIS AND STEPHANIA COMBINATION

2.0 Tang-kuei	Danggui	LV; nourishes and vitalizes Blood
2.0 Peony	Baishao	
2.0 Cnidium	Chuanxiong	
2.0 Rehmannia	Dihuang	
1.5 Siler	Fangfeng	LU/BL; dispels wind, relieves pain
1.5 Chin-chiu	Qinjiao	
1.0 Angelica	Baizhi	
1.5 Chiang-huo	Qianghuo	
1.5 Clematis	Weilingxian	
1.5 Ginger	Shengjiang	
1.5 Stephania	Fangji	BL; clears moisture
2.0 Hoelen	Fuling	
1.5 Citrus	Chenpi	SP; tonifies Chi
2.0 Atractylodes	Baizhu	
1.0 Licorice	Gancao	

NOTES:

折衝飲

CINNAMON AND PERSICA COMBINATION

Che Cung Yin

LITERAL: Break the Blockage Special Remedy

THERAPEUTIC PRINCIPLES: dispel stagnant Blood, relieve pain.

INDICATIONS: severe menstrual pain, postpartum pain, endometriosis, uterine tumor.

PULSE: congested, knotty, fast

TONGUE: may have purplish spots

HERBS AND ACTIONS: Carthamus, achyranthes, persica, moutan, cnidium, peony, tang-kuei, and corydalis all dispel stagnant Blood and relieve pain; cinnamon opens the Blood channels; tang-kuei, peony, and cnidium also nourish the production of new Blood.

TYPICAL VARIATIONS: For constipation, add rhubarb; for general weakness, add codonopsis, alisma, hoelen, and white atractylodes; for low back pain and for endometriosis, add dipsacus; for cold hands/feet and facial flushing, add bupleurum, chih-ko, and licorice; for scanty menstruation and pre-menstrual syndrome, add saussurea (this will produce **Achyranthes Formula** with carthamus and cnidium added).

4.0 Persica	Taoren	LV; vitalizes Blood
3.0 Cnidium	Chuanxiong	
3.0 Achyranthes	Niuxi	
3.0 Corydalis	Yanhusuo	
1.0 Carthamus	Honghua	
5.0 Tang-kuei	Danggui	LV; tonifies and vitalizes Blood
3.0 Peony	Baishao	

3.0 Moutan	Mudanpi	LV; cools and vitalizes Blood
3.0 Cinnamon	Guizhi	servant; opens vessels

NOTES:

仙方活命飲

ANGELICA AND MASTIC COMBINATION

Xian Fang Huo Ming Yin

LITERAL: The Immortals' Special Prescription for Long Life

THERAPEUTIC PRINCIPLES: activate Blood circulation, dispel wind, clean toxin, clear phlegm and pus.

INDICATIONS: tumors, swellings, skin eruptions and other accumulations and hard masses.

PULSE: rapid, knotty

TONGUE: may have purplish areas; coated

HERBS AND ACTIONS: Anteater scales, myrrh, mastic, tang-kuei, and peony activate circulation of Blood; angelica and siler dispel wind and relieve pain; gleditsia spine, fritillaria, and trichosanthes root clear phlegm and dispel pus; lonicera cleans toxins; citrus activates circulation of Chi.

TYPICAL VARIATIONS: For more severe toxic syndrome, add forsythia and houtteynia; for more severe inflammation, add coptis and phellodendron; for stronger wind-dispelling action, add schizonepeta and mentha.

3.0 Anteater scales	Chuanshanjia	LV; vitalizes Blood
3.0 Myrrh	Muyao	
3.0 Mastic	Ruxiang	
3.0 Tang-kuei	Danggui	LV; nourishes and vitalizes Blood
3.0 Peony	Baishao	
3.0 Angelica	Baizhi	LU; dispels wind
3.0 Siler	Fangfeng	
3.0 Gleditsia spine	Zaojaioci	LU; clears heated phlegm
3.0 Trichosanthes root	Tianhuafen	
3.0 Fritillaria	Zhibeimu	

ANGELICA AND MASTIC COMBINATION

9.0 Lonicera	Jinyinhua	HT; cleans toxins
9.0 Citrus	Chenpi	SP; disperses Chi
3.0 Licorice	Gancao	servant; harmonizer

NOTES:

芎歸調血飲

CNIDIUM AND REHMANNIA COMBINATION

Xiong Gui Tiao Xue Yin

LITERAL: Cnidium and Tang-kuei Circulate Blood Special Formula

THERAPEUTIC PRINCIPLES: vitalize circulation of Chi and Blood; tonify Chi and Blood.

INDICATIONS: menstrual disorders, menopausal syndrome, postpartum disorders, abdominal pains, emotional distress.

PULSE: thin, weak, wiry

TONGUE: pale; may have purple spots

HERBS AND ACTIONS: Leonorus, tang-kuei, cnidium, and moutan vitalize circulation of blood; rehmannia, tang-kuei, and cnidium nourish Blood; hoelen, atractylodes, ginger, licorice, and jujube benefit digestion and tonify Chi; lindera, cyperus, and citrus disperse stagnant Chi and relieve emotional distress.

TYPICAL VARIATIONS: This is a large **Ming Dynasty formula** and is usually not modified. For more severe abdominal pains, add achyranthes and salvia or red peony; for insomnia and nightsweating of menopause, add gelatin and astragalus; for neurotic symptoms, add perilla leaf, longan, and pinellia.

1.5 Leonorus	Yimucao	LV; vitalizes Blood
2.0 Moutan	Mudanpi	
2.0 Cnidium	Chuanxiong	
2.0 Lindera	Wuyao	LV/SP; vitalizes Chi
2.0 Cyperus	Xiangfu	
2.0 Citrus	Chenpi	

CNIDIUM AND REHMANNIA COMBINATION

2.0 Tang-kuei	Danggui	LV/nourishes Blood
2.0 Rehmannia	Dihuang	
2.0 Atractylodes	Baizhu	SP/ST; normalizes digestion, tonifies Chi
2.0 Hoelen	Fuling	
1.5 Licorice	Gancao	
1.5 Jujube	Dazao	
1.5 Ginger	Ganjiang	

NOTES:

INTRODUCTION TO MOISTURE MOVING HERBS

Moisture usually accumulates as a result of dysfunctions of the Kidney, Spleen, and Lung. Hoelen is the main moisture resolving herb and is usually combined with herbs that direct it to the organ system most responsible for the problem in moving moisture.

Moisture moving formulas are also used for the treatment of inflammations of the urogenital tract, usually by including cold-energy moisture-moving herbs and other fire purging herbs.

Moisture problems often show up as:

edema
bladder infection
swelling of joints
diarrhea
headaches
soft pulse
kidney inflammation
change in urinary frequency
digestive weakness
watery blisters
heart palpitations
swollen tongue

STANDARD MATCHING IN MOISTURE MOVING FORMULAS

HOELEN AND ATRACTYLODES: relieves digestive upset, diarrhea, and abdominal bloating.

POLYPORUS AND ALISMA: treats nephritis and urinary tract disorders.

TALC AND GELATIN: relieves urinary tract bleeding and burning

ACONITE AND GINGER: clear moisture related to a syndrome of internal cold.

CAUTIONS ABOUT MOISTURE MOVING FORMULAS

It is rare that a moisture moving formula will cause any adverse reaction; however, if the prescription is not correct for the individual, symptoms that are usually treated by these formulas may arise. If the person suffers from a dryness condition, the Moisture moving formula may exacerbate the condition.

真武湯

VITALITY COMBINATION

Chen Wu Tang

LITERAL: True Martial Decoction

THERAPEUTIC PRINCIPLES: dispels chills, moves dampness, strengthens Yang.

INDICATIONS: chills, aversion to cold, diarrhea, abdominal bloating, weakness, indigestion, loss of hair, fatigue, surface pains.

PULSE: weak

TONGUE: pale, moist; white or grey fur

HERBS AND ACTIONS: Aconite, ginger, and atractylodes dispel chills, strengthen the Kidney, Spleen, and Heart, and move Moisture; hoelen helps move Moisture; peony harmonizes the Ying and Wei Chi; aconite with peony relieves surface pain.

TYPICAL VARIATIONS: For chronic weak digestion, add codonopsis; for night sweats, add astragalus; for prolapse of organs, add astragalus and codonopsis; for severe body aches, add cinnamon twig; for severe internal chill and intestinal colic, add zanthoxylum; for lower body weakness, add fennel, achyranthes, and eucommia; for chronic diarrhea, add dioscorea and lotus seed; for weak pulse and for asthmatic breathing induced by cold, add ginseng, schizandra, and ophiopogon (this will produce **Vitality Combination** with **Ginseng, Schizandra, and Ophiopogon Combination**); for ulcer and water accumulation in the Stomach, add pinellia, jujube, cinnamon, and licorice (this will produce **Hoelen and Jujube Combination** with aconite and atractylodes); for ulcer with pyloric obstruction, add alisma, cinnamon, and licorice (this will produce **Alisma and Hoelen Combination** with peony and aconite); for edema with general aching and diarrhea, add ginseng (this will produce **Aconite Combination** with ginger added); for monoplagiea or arthritis with severe chills, add cinnamon, jujube, and licorice (this will produce **Cinnamon and Atractylodes Combination**); for weakness of the legs and joint swelling, add cinnamon, siler, annemarhena, Ma-huang and licorice (this will produce **Cinnamon and Anemarrhena Combination** with hoelen added).

5.0 Hoelen	Fuling	SP; moves Moisture
3.0 Atractylodes	Baizhu	
3.0 Ginger	Ganjiang	SP/KI; dispels chill,
1.0 Aconite	Fuzi	moisture
3.0 Peony	Baishao	LV; relieves spasm

NOTES:

五苓散

HOELEN FIVE HERB FORMULA

Wu Ling San

THERAPEUTIC PRINCIPLES: move Moisture, strengthen Kidney and Spleen.

INDICATIONS: diarrhea, abdominal bloating, general weakness, change in urinary frequency, emotional instability, mild edema.

PULSE: floating and fast

TONGUE: some moist, thin white coating

HERBS AND ACTIONS: Cinnamon twig with hoelen relieves surface Moisture; with alisma, hoelen nourishes the Spleen; alisma, polyporus, and hoelen are diuretics, strengthen Kidney and relieve edema.

TYPICAL VARIATIONS: For Liver/Spleen disharmony and for half-inside, half-surface disorders, add **Minor Bupleurum Combination** (this will produce **Bupleurum and Hoelen Combination**); for urinary burning or bleeding, add talc and gelatin; for nausea and vomiting, add ginger and pinellia; for jaundice, add capillaris (this will produce **Capillaris and Hoelen Formula**), for arthralgia with general edema (especially lower body), add siler, Chiang-huo, and codonopsis; for abdominal bloating and weakness, add magnolia bark, citrus, and **Cinnamon Combination** (this will produce **Magnolia and Hoelen Combination** with peony added); for heart palpitations, insomnia, or gastric ulcer, add saussurea, coptis, and ginger (this will produce **Hoelen and Saussurea Combination**).

4.5 Hoelen	Fuling	SP/KI; moves moisture
4.5 Alisma	Zexie	
4.5 Polyporus	Zhuling	
4.5 Atracylodes	Baizhu	SP/ST; moves moisture

3.0 Cinnamon	Guizhi	servant; opens vessels

NOTES:

防已黃耆湯

STEPHANIA AND ASTRAGALUS COMBINATION

Fang Ji Huang Chi Tang

THERAPEUTIC PRINCIPLES: relieve inflammation, clear moisture.

INDICATIONS: pain in the knees and legs, edema of the legs, abdominal bloating.

PULSE: floating, weak

TONGUE: swollen, moist

HERBS AND ACTIONS: Stephania relieves inflammation, and with atractylodes and astragalus clears excess moisture; ginger, licorice, and jujube are servants that enhance Chi.

TYPICAL VARIATIONS: For more severe edema, add hoelen and cinnamon twig (this will produce **Stephania and Hoelen Combination** with atractylodes, giriger, and jujube added); for hypertension, add salvia; for reduced urination or painful urination, add talc; for arthritis, add siler, tu-huo, and hoelen.

5.0 Stephania	Fangji	Lung/Bladder; circulates moisture
5.0 Astragalus	Huangqi	Spleen; tonifies Chi
3.0 Atractylodes	Baizhu	
3.0 Ginger	Ganjiang	servants
1.5 Licorice	Gancao	
3.0 Jujube	Dazao	

猪苓湯

POLYPORUS COMBINATION

Zhu Ling Tang

THERAPEUTIC PRINCIPLES: promote diuresis, relieve inflammation, stop bleeding.

INDICATIONS: painful urination, prostatic inflammation, nephritis, kidney gravel, diarrhea.

PULSE: rapid, floating

TONGUE: yellow coating at back of tongue

HERBS AND ACTIONS: Polyporus, hoelen, alisma, and talc all promote diuresis and relieve inflammation of the urinary tract; gelatin helps stop bleeding due to inflammation.

TYPICAL VARIATIONS: For more severe inflammation and for accompanying constipation, add gardenia; for deficient urination, add cooked rehmannia; for general weakness and digestive disturbance, add atractylodes; for chronic prostatic inflammation, add polygonum, dianthus, and akebia; for diarrhea, add dioscorea and codonopsis.

3.0 Polyporus	Zhuling	KI/BL; moves Moisture, purges fire
3.0 Hoelen	Fuling	
3.0 Alisma	Zexie	
3.0 Talc	Huashi	
3.0 Gelatin	Ejiao	KI; arrests bleeding, tonifies Yin

半夏厚朴湯

PINELLIA AND MAGNOLIA COMBINATION

Ban Xia Hou Pu Tang

THERAPEUTIC PRINCIPLES: disperse stagnant Chi, Moisture, and Phlegm.

INDICATIONS: plumpit Chi syndrome, nausea, vomiting, morning sickness, abdominal bloating, bronchitis.

PULSE: floating and weak, or sinking and thin

TONGUE: moist, swollen

HERBS AND ACTIONS: Perilla leaf and magnolia bark disperse stagnant Chi and Moisture; hoelen aids in moving Moisture; pinellia and ginger help clear phlegm.

TYPICAL VARIATIONS: For tightness of the chest and coughing, add platycodon, bupleurum, morus, and apricot seed (this will produce **Aurantium and Pinellia Combination** with cyperus and aurantium deleted); for ulcer, add ginseng, cinnamon, scute, and licorice (this will produce **Hoelen and Pinellia Combination** with perilla added) or add only ginseng and licorice (this will produce **Magnolia Five Combination** with perilla and hoelen added).

6.0 Pinellia	Banxia	SP/ST; resolves phlegm
4.0 Ginger	Ganjiang	
2.0 Perilla	Zisuye	SP; circulates Chi
3.0 Magnolia bark	Houpu	and Moisture
5.0 Hoelen	Fuling	SP; moves Moisture

半夏白朮天麻湯

PINELLIA AND GASTRODIA COMBINATION

Ban Xia Bai Zhu Tien Ma Tang

THERAPEUTIC PRINCIPLES: clear congestion, move Moisture, dissolve phlegm, tonify Chi.

INDICATIONS: fullness after eating, headaches, sinus congestion, food allergy.

PULSE: weak, rapid, sinking

TONGUE: greasy coating; tongue may be swollen

HERBS AND ACTIONS: Shen-chu and malt clear congestion of stagnant food; pinellia, citrus, ginger, hoelen, and alisma clear dampness and phlegm; astragalus, ginseng, and atractylodes tonify Chi; phellodendron clears heat; gastrodia calms internal wind and relieves headaches.

TYPICAL VARIATIONS: For headaches, add angelica; for indigestion, add crataegus; for shoulder/neck tension, add pueraria; for symptoms of heated phlegm, add bamboo; for abdominal pain, add cardamon and saussurea.

2.0 Shen-chu	Shenqu	SP/ST; clears undigested food
2.0 Malt	Maiya	
1.5 Alisma	Zexie	SP/ST; moves Moisture
3.5 Hoelen	Fuling	
1.5 Ginseng	Renshen	SP/ST; tonifies Chi
1.5 Astragalus	Huangqi	
3.0 Atractylodes	Baizhu	
3.0 Pinellia	Banxia	SP/ST; clears Moisture and Phlegm
3.0 Citrus	Chenpi	
2.0 Ginger	Ganjiang	
2.0 Gastrodia	Tianma	LV; sedates internal wind
1.0 Phellodendron	Huangbai	LI; clears heat and dampness

二陳湯

CITRUS AND PINELLIA COMBINATION

Er Chen Tang

LITERAL: Two Aged Substances Decoction

THERAPEUTIC PRINCIPLES: clear dampness and phlegm; warm the Gallbladder.

INDICATIONS: nausea, vomiting, diarrhea, excessive sputum production, headache, hangover.

PULSE: slippery to soft

TONGUE: moist to greasy coating; tongue may be swollen

HERBS AND ACTIONS: This formula is made from **Minor Pinellia and Hoelen Combination** by adding citrus and licorice. Hoelen clears excess moisture; pinellia dissolves phlegm; citrus clears both moisture and phlegm; ginger and licorice promote digestive functions and thereby reduce accumulations of moisture.

TYPICAL VARIATIONS: For weakness of Chi, add ginseng, atractylodes, and jujube (this will produce **Six Major Herbs Combination**); for insomnia and heart palpitations, add chih-shih, bamboo, coptis, and zizyphus (this will produce **Bamboo and Hoelen Combination**); for ulcer and gastric distress, add magnolia bark, atractylodes (cangzhu), and jujube (this will produce **Magnolia and Ginger Formula** with hoelen and pinellia added) or add magnolia bark, ginseng, cinnamon, and scute (this will produce **Hoelen and Pinellia Combination** with citrus added); for diarrhea and abdominal pain related to stagnant food, add crataegus, Shen-chu, raphanus, and forsythia (this will produce **Citrus and Crataegus Formula** with pinellia and ginger added); for plumpit Chi syndrome and for morning sickness, add magnolia bark and perilla leaf (this will produce **Pinellia and Magnolia Combination** with citrus and licorice added); for food poisoning and summer heat syndrome, add atractylodes, magnolia bark, agastache, and jujube (this will produce **Pinellia, Atractylodes, and Agastache Formula**); for acute gastric distress with diarrhea and vomiting, add ginseng, aconite, coptis, and jujube (this will produce **Pinellia and Jujube Combination** with citrus added).

4.0 Citrus	Chenpi	SP/ST; clears Moisture, normalizes digestion
5.0 Pinellia	Banxia	
5.0 Hoelen	Fuling	
3.0 Ginger	Ganjiang	
1.0 Licorice	Gancao	

NOTES:

SINGLE HERBS SUBSTITUTION GUIDE

Every herb in the Chinese pharmacopeia is unique, yet the herbs can be subsumed under major categories according to their principal therapeutic effects. A typical listing of Chinese herbs will be presented in about thirty categories. Within a category, there are notable differences among the herbs, but there are certain herbs that are particularly close to each other in properties and those are the ones most easily used in substitution.

When producing a personalized formula, it may happen that one or two of the herbs called for in the recipe are not available at the time. Depending upon the size of the formula and the significance of the missing herbs, the herbs might simply be deleted, or they might be replaced by other herbs.

Below are some examples of herbs that might be interchanged in the event that the desired one is not available or is too costly:

WARM WIND DISPELLING: siler, chiang-huo, tu-huo
COLD WIND DISPELLING: morus leaf, chrysanthemum
PURGATIVE: rhubarb, gardenia
FIRE PURGING: rehmannia (raw), scrophularia
PURGE FIRE, DRY DAMPNESS: coptis, scute, phellodendron;
CHILL DISPELLING: cinnamon bark, aconite
FRAGRANT MOISTURE RESOLVING: cardamon, cluster
CHI REGULATING: aquilaria, lindera
HEMOSTATIC: sanguisorba, bulrush (fried pollen typhae)
BLOOD VITALIZING (cold energy): salvia, red peony, moutan

BLOOD VITALIZING (warm energy): zedoria, turmeric, myrrh, mastic
CHI TONICS: ginseng, codonopsis, pseudostellaria
YANG TONICS: eucommia, dispacus
YIN TONICS: glehnia, American ginseng
ASTRINGENTS: schizandra, mume
HEAVY SEDATIVES: oyster shell, dragon bone
PHLEGM RESOLVING: laminaria, sargassum
CONGESTION RESOLVING: malt, oryza

There are numerous other examples that can be selected. To choose a substitute, the most important factor is matching the desired therapeutic action. Thus, whether or not the herbs are in the same section of the Chinese pharmacopeia or of the same energy can be secondary to the concern for principal effect of the herb. In some cases, two herbs may be used as a substitute for one herb in order to match the desired action.

In general, herbs that are frequently used together within formulas are the herbs that can substitute for one another. The inclusion of herbs of similar action within a formula is one in which the herbalist reinforces the action of each herb. Thus, the pairs myrrh and mastic, laminaria and sargassum, coptis and scute, cinnamon and aconite, oyster shell and dragon bone, cardamom and cluster are commonly found in traditional prescriptions with each member of the pair having very similar activities.

Substitution is much easier when the herb is used as an adjunct rather than as the primary herb. Hence, for dredging the Chi of the Liver and relieving liver tension, bupleurum is often used as the primary herb. It is difficult to replace in formulas such as Minor Bupleurum Combination, Bupleurum and Peony Formula, and Bupleurum and Dragon Bone Combination. However, as an adjunct therapy, it can be substituted as a surface relieving herb by cimicifuga or pueraria, as an herb to raise the Chi and Yang by cimicifuga, or as an herb to regulate menstruation by curcuma.

In short formulas, comprised of not more than eight herbs, it is more difficult to make substitutions because of the relatively large impact of each herb in the formula. In such cases, it is important to closely match the taste and energetic impact (e.g. dispersing or consolidating, moisturizing or drying; bitter/purging or sweet/tonifying). Very often, these short formulas are carefully harmonized by balancing the impact of one herb with that on another. Ginger and jujube, cinnamon twig and peony, coptis and cinnamon bark, schizandra and ophiopogon, are examples of the herbs that are paired up to produce the desired effect.

In larger formulas, one need only approximate the impact of the herb according to these parameters. Thus, Ho-shou-wu and lycium fruit are both tonics to the Blood, Yin, and Essence and can be combined or substituted for one another if one needs such a tonic in a large formula. However, Ho-shou-wu is a bitter, warm astringent, while lycium fruit is a sweet, neutral, moist herb; in this sense, their properties are quite different. Ho-shou-wu is suitable for treating leukorrhea and intestinal disorders for which lycium fruit is not suitable.

In some cases, a single herb which is to be used as an addition to a formula can be substituted by a short combination of herbs. For example, coptis is often added to prescriptions in order to purge Heart fire or to treat a damp heat syndrome (dysentery, skin disorders, membrane inflammation). However, the herb is quite expensive and its effects are reproduced very well by the Coptis and Scute Combination. This combination contains four herbs, all of which are helpful in purging fire and drying dampness. The three herbs combined with coptis are much less expensive than coptis alone. Similarly, ginseng is often prescribed for restoring Chi, benefiting digestion, and as an adjunct to Blood tonics (such as Tang-kuei). This herb is also quite expensive and is sometimes substituted by codonopsis. However, codonopsis has a weaker effect on persons with severely debilitated Chi. Instead, one might use Four Major Herbs Combination, which as a formula has effects similar to those of ginseng, one of its ingredients. The combination of four herbs is much less expensive than ginseng. In like manner, Tang-kuei Four Combination might be used in place of the single herb Tang-kuei; Vitality Combination could be used in place of the single herb aconite.

The idea of combining therapeutic principles rather than individual herbs is one of the unique and important aspects of Chinese medicine. According to this way of thinking, it is not a specific herb, or drug, that is called for, but a certain approach to harmonizing the body. Certainly, some herbs will work out better for one patient or another, but this is something that is difficult to predict in advance. Because one is working with a wholistic approach to health care, it should not be the particular herb or formula that is critical, but rather the ability to encourage the body in the direction of the healthy balance point.

INDEX OF HERB NAMES

COMMON NAME	PINYIN	PHARMACEUTICAL NAME
achyranthes	niuxi	radix achyranthis bidentatae
aconite	fuzi	radix aconiti carmichaeli praeparata
acorus	changpu	rhizoma acori graminei
agastache	huoxiang	herba agastaches rugosa
akebia	mutong	caulis akebiae
alisma	zexie	rhizoma alismatis
anemarrhena	zhimu	rhizoma anemarrhenae
angelica	baizhi	radix angelicae dahurica
anteater scale	chuanshanjia	squama manitis
apricot seed	xingren	semen armeniacae amarae
aquilaria	chenxiang	lignum aquilariae
arctium	niubangzi	fructus arctii
areca seed	binglangzi	semen arecae
arisaema	tiannanxing	rhizoma arisaematis
artemisia	aiye	folium artemisiae argyi
asarum	xixin	herba asari cum radice
asparagus	tianmendong	radix asparagi
aster	ziwan	radix asteris
astragalus	huangqi	radix astragali
atractylodes (b)	cangzhu	rhizoma atracylodis lanceae
atractylodes (w)	baizhu	rhizoma atractylodis alba
aurantium	jupi	exocarpium aurantii
bamboo	zhuru	caulis bambussae in taeniis
benincasa	dongguazi	semen benincasae
biota	boziren	semen biotae
broussonetia	chushizi	fructus broussonetiae
bupleurum	chaihu	radix bupleuri
cannabis (linum)	huomaren	semen cannabis
capillaris	yinchenhao	herba artemesiae capillaris
cardamon	suosha	fructus seu semen amomi
carthamus	honghua	flos carthami
cassia seed	huemingzi	semen cassiae torae

COMMON NAME	PINYIN	PHARMACEUTICAL NAME
chaenomeles	mugua	fructus chaenomelis lagenariae
chiang-huo	qianghuo	rhizoma et radix notopterygii
chih-ko	zhiko	fructus aurantii
chih-shih	zhishi	fructus aurantii immaturus
chrysanthemum	juhua	flos chrysanthemi
cicada	chantui	periostracum cicadae
cimicifuga	shengma	rhizoma cimicifugae
cinnamon bark	guipi	cortex cinnamoni
cinnamon twigs	guizhi	ramulus cinnamomi
cistanche	roucongrong	herba cistanchis
citrus	chenpi	expcarpum citri leiocarpae
clematis	weilingxian	radix clematidis
cnidium	chuanxiong	radix ligustici wallichii
codonopsis	dangshen	radix codonopsis pilosulae
coix	yiyiren	semen coicis
coptis	huanglian	rhizoma coptidis
cornus	shanzhuyu	fructus corni
corydalis	yanhusuo	rhizoma corydalis
crataegus	shanzha	fructus crataegi
curcuma	jianghuang	radix curcumae
cuscuta	tusizi	semen cuscutae
cyperus	xiangfuzi	rhizoma cyperi
dendrobium	shihu	herba dendrobii
dioscorea	shanyao	radix dioscorea batatis
dipsacus	xuduan	radix dipsaci
dolichos seed	baipiandou	semen dolichoris
dragon bone	longgu	os draconis
eclipta	hanliancao	herba ecliptae
elsholtzia	xiangru	herba elsholtziae
epimedium	yinyanghuo	herba epimedii
eriobotrya	pipaye	folium eriobotryae
eucommia	duzhong	cortex eucommiae
euryale	qianshi	semen euryalis
evodia	wuzhuyu	fructus evodiae
figwort	xuanshen	radix scrophulariae
forsythia	lianqiao	fructus forsythiae
fritillaria	beimu	bulbus fritillariae
gambir (uncaria)	diaotenggou	ramulus uncariae cum uncus

COMMON NAME	PINYIN	PHARMACEUTICAL NAME
gardenia	zhizi	fructus gardenia
gastrodia	tianma	rhizoma gastrodiae
gelatin	ajiao	asini gelatinum
gentiana	longdan	radix gentianae scabrae
ginger (dry)	ganjiang	rhizoma zingiberis siccatum
ginseng	renshen	radix ginseng
gleditsia	zaoci	spina gleditsiae
gypsum	shigao	gypsum fibrosum
haliotis	shijueming	concha haliotidis
hoelen	fuling	poria cocos
inula	xuanfuhua	flos inulae
jujube	dazao	fructus zizyphi sativae
juncus	dengxincao	medulla junci
laminaria	haidai	herba laminaria
lashiosphaera	mabo	rhizoma lashiosphaera
leonurus	yimucao	herba leonuri
licorice	gancao	radix glycyrrhizae
lily	baihe	bulbus lilii
lindera	wuyao	radix linderae
linum	maziren	semen cannabis
lithospermum	zicao	radix macrotomiae seu lithospermi
longan	lungyenrou	arillus longanae
lonicera	jinyinhua	flos lonicerae
loranthus	sangjisheng	ramulus loranthi
lotus seed	lianzi	semen nelumbinis
lycium fruit	gouqizi	fructus lycii
lycium bark	digupi	cortex lycii radicis
magnolia bark	houpu	cortex magnoliae officinalis
magnolia flower	xinyi	flos magnoliae liliflorae
ma-huang	mahuang	herba ephedra
mastic	ruxiang	gumni olibanum
melia	chuanlianzi	fructus meliae toosendan
mentha	bohe	herba menthae
mirabilitum	mangxiao	magnesii sulfuricum
morinda	bajitian	radix morindae
morus leaf	sangye	folium mori
morus bark	sanghaipi	cortex mori radicis
moutan	mudanpi	cortex moutan radicis

COMMON NAME	PINYIN	PHARMACEUTICAL NAME
mume	wumei	fructus mume
myrrh	moyao	myrrha
ophiopogon	maimendong	radix ophiopogonis
oryza	guya	fructus oryzae germinatus
oyster shell	muli	concha ostreae
peony	shaoyao	radix paeoniae alba
perilla seed	zisuzi	semen perillae frutescentis
perilla leaf	zisuye	folium perillae acutae
perilla fruit	zisuzi	fructus perillae frutescentis
persica	taoren	semen persicae
peucedanum	qianhu	radix peucedani
phellodendron	huangbo	cortex phellodendri
phragmites	lugen	rhizoma phragmitis
pinellia	banxia	rhizoma pinelliae
plantago	cheqianzi	semen plataginis
platycodon	jiegeng	radix platycodi
polygala	yuanzhi	radix polygalae
polygonatum	yuzhu	rhizoma polygonati officinalis
polygonum	heshouwu	radix polygoni multiflori
polyporus	zhuling	polyporus
prunella	xiakucao	spica prunellae
psoralea	buguzhi	fructus psoraleae
pueraria	gegen	radix puerariae
rehmannia (cooked)	shudihuang	radix rehmanniae (cooked)
rehmannia (raw)	shengdihuang	radix rehmanniae (raw)
red peony	chishao	radix paeoniae rubra
rhubarb	dahuang	rhizoma rhei
salvia	danshen	radix salviae miltiorrhizae
saussurea	muxiang	radix saussureae
schizandra	wuweizi	fructus schizandrae
schizonepeta	jingjie	herba schizonepetae
scrophularia	xuanshen	radix scrophulariae
scute	huangqin	radix scutellariae
sesame	humaren	semen sesami
siler	fangfeng	radix ledebouriellae
silkworm	baijiangcan	bombyx mori
soja	dandouchi	semen sojae praeparatum

COMMON NAME	PINYIN	PHARMACEUTICAL NAME
sophora	kushen	radix sophorae flavescentis
stephania	fangchi	radix stephania tetranda
succinum	hupo	succinum
talc	huashi	talcum
tang-kuei	danggui	radix angelicae sinensis
tribulus	jili	fructus tribuli
trichosanthes root	gualougen	radix trichosanthis
trichosanthes seed	gualouren	semen trichosanthis
tu-huo	duhuo	radix angelicae tuhuo
tussilago	kuandonghua	flos farfarae
vitex	manjingzi	fructus viticis
zanthoxylum	shanjiao	fructus zanthoxyli
zedoaria	ezhu	rhizoma zedoariae
zizyphus	suanzaoren	semen zizyphi spinosae

INDEX OF SYMPTOMS AND SIGNS

Chinese herb prescribing is usually done according to symptom complex, or conformation. This means that one takes into account many aspects of the person's health, looks for a basic pattern, and then prescribes accordingly. The basic patterns one looks for are congruent with the indications for the traditional herb formulas; one then modifies the formulas, if necessary, to bring them more into line with the person's specific condition.

Experienced Chinese doctors generally know, after examining a patient, which of the many traditional formulas are applicable, having memorized both the ingredients and indications for them.

Newer practitioners often must spend some time examining written explanations of the formulas (such as provided in this book), in order to determine whether or not they approximately match the patient's needs. To assist the practitioner in looking up formulas in this book, the following symptoms index is provided. For each symptom or disease, one or more formulas is recommended as a starting point. This formula should not be chosen, however, unless the description fits the patient reasonably well. If not, consider other formulas in the same section of the book, or return to this index and look for other symptoms that are of similar nature or affecting a similar area of the body for other suggestions of herb formulas.

Formulas that fit the general needs of the patient may successfully relieve symptoms which are not mentioned when the formula is described. This is because there are many possible symptomatic outcomes of the same underlying imbalance.

Use the symptoms of predominant concern for guidance in the index below. To make the process of symptom selection easier, they have been divided here by parts of the body, starting at the top and working down, followed by an index of mental symptoms and miscellaneous items.

HEAD:

Acne . . . . Bupleurum and Schizonepeta

Bitter taste	Minor Bupleurum Combination
Cold/flu	Lonicera and Forsythia Formula, Pueraria Combination
Dandruff (dry scalp)	Tang-kuei and Arctium Combination
Ear infections	Scute and Cimicufuga Combination
Eye infections	Gardenia and Vitex Combination
Eye redness, swelling	Coptis and Scute Combination
Facial flushing	Rehmannia Six Formula
Headache	Ophiopogon and Asarum Combination, Gambir Formula
Hearing problems	Rehmannia Six Formula
Jaw tension	Bupleurum Formula
Loss of Hair	Lycium Formula, Ginseng Nutritive Combination
Nose bleed	Coptis and Scute Combination
Shoulder/neck tension	Bupleurum and Cinnamon Combination/Pueraria Comb.
Sinus problems	Pueraria Nasal Combination, Magnolia and Gypsum Comb.
Sore throat	Cimicifuga and Scute Combination
Swollen glands	Bupleurum and Rehmannia Combination
Thirst	Gypsum Combination
Tongue inflammation	Cnidium and Moutan Combination
Trigeminal neuralgia	Ophiopogon and Asarum Combination

CHEST:

Asthma	Ma-huang and Ginkgo, Minor Blue Dragon Combination
Breast lumps, swelling	Bupleurum and Cyperus; Tang-kuei Sixteen Herb Comb.
Bronchitis	Bupleurum, Cinnamon, and Ginger Combination
Cold/flu	Ma-huang and Morus Combination

Coughing, copious sputum . . Platycodon and Fritillaria Combination
Coughing, dry . . . . Lily Combination, Ophiopogon Combination
Heart palpitations . . . . Ginseng and Zizyphus Combination
Intercostal neuralgia . . . . Minor Bupleurum Combination
Lung heat . . . . Bupleurum and Ginseng, Phellodendron Combination
Pneumonia . . . . Bupleurum and Pueraria Combination

MID SECTION:

Digestive disturbance . . . . . . Six Major Herbs Combination
Food allergy . . . . Minor Bupleurum Combination
Gallbladder disorders . . . . . . Major Bupleurum; Bupleurum and Chih-shih Combination
Hepatitis . . . . Minor Bupleurum Combination
Indigestion . . . . Pinellia and Gastrodia Combination
Liver cirrhosis . . . . Bupleurum and Peony Formula
Loss of appetite . . . . Four Major Herbs Combination
Morning sickness . . . . Pinellia and Magnolia Combination
Nausea . . . . Citrus and Pinellia Combination
Pancreatic inflammation . . . . Pinellia Combination, Minor Bupleurum Combination
Stomachache . . . . Bupleurum and Evodia Combination
Subcostal bloating . . . . Bupleurum and Magnolia Combination
Ulcer . . . . Bupleurum and Evodia; Minor Bupleurum Combination
Vomiting . . . . Pinellia Combination
Weak digestion . . . . Four Major Herbs Combination

INTESTINES:

Blockage, masses . . . . Bupleurum and Pinellia Combination
Colitis . . . . Bupleurum and Cinnamon Combination

Constipation (acute) . . . . Minor Rhubarb Combination
Diarrhea, enteritis . . . . Pinellia Combination

WAIST AND PELVIS:

Bloating . . . . Cinnamon and Hoelen Combination
Dysmenorrhea . . . . Cinnamon and Persica Combination
Genital herpes . . . . Gentiana Combination
Impotence . . . . Lycium Formula
Infertility (female) . . . . Ginseng and Tang-kuei Ten Combination
Leukorrhea . . . . Ginseng and Longan Combination
Low back ache . . . . Tang-kuei and Rehmannia Combination
Menstrual irregularity . . . . . . Cnidium and Rehmannia Combination
Pelvic inflammatory disease . . Moutan and Persica Combination
Urinary tract infection . . . . . . Polyporus Combination
Vaginal infection . . . . Bupleurum and Peony Formula

LIMBS:

Arthritis . . . . Cinnamon and Anemarrhena; Major Siler; Coix; Tang-kuei and Anemarrhena; Clematis and Stephania
Cold Hands/Feet . . . . Bupleurum and Chih-shih Combination
Coordination problems . . . . . Bupleurum and Dragon Bone Combination
Gout . . . . Clematis and Stephania Combination
Knee swelling . . . . Stephania and Astragalus Combination
Knee weakness . . . . Lycium Formula
Muscular weakness . . . . Major Siler Combination
Neuralgia . . . . Clematis and Stephania Combination

Numbness . . . . Vitality Combination, Cinnamon and Anemarrhnea Comb.
Paralysis . . . . Cinnamon and Anemarrhena, Major Siler Combination
Rheumatism . . . . Coix Combination
Sciatica . . . . Clematis and Stephania Combination

MENTAL CONDITIONS:

Amnesia . . . . Ginseng and Longan Combination
Depression . . . . Bupleurum and Cyperus, Bupleurum and Peony Formula
Emotional instability . . . . Bamboo and Ginseng Combination
Insomnia . . . . Ginseng and Zizyphus; Bupleurum and Dragon Bone Combination
Irritability, Nervousness . . . . . Bupleurum and Dragon Bone; Bupleurum Formula
Neurosis . . . . Ginseng and Zizyphus Combination
Withdrawal syndrome . . . . . . Bupleurum and Dragon Bone Combination

OTHER:

Alcoholism . . . . Bupleurum and Dragon Bone; Bupleurum and Peony Formula
Anemia . . . . Ginseng and Tang-kuei Ten; Tang-kuei Four, Ginseng and Longan Combination
Boils . . . . Coptis and Scute; Siler and Platycodon Combination
Chills . . . . Vitality Combination
Chiropractic . . . . Bupleurum and Cinnamon Combination
Diabetes . . . . Rehmannia Six Formula, Phellodendron Combination
Dry skin . . . . Tang-kuei and Arctium; Tang-kuei Four Combination

Eczema . . . . Tang-kuei and Arctium Combination
Edema . . . . Bupleurum and Magnolia; Hoelen Five Herb Formula
Epilepsy . . . . Bupleurum and Cinnamon Combination
Feverish feeling . . . . Astragalus and Atractylodes Combination
General Weakness . . . . Ginseng Nutritive Combination
Hypertension . . . . Siler and Platycodon Combination
Hypoglycemia . . . . Bupleurum and Cinnamon Combination
Immune system weakness . . . Ginseng and Longan; Astragalus and Atractylodes, Ginseng Nutritive Combination
Itchy/burning skin . . . . Tang-kuei and Arctium Combination
Low body weight . . . . Four Major Herbs Combination
Lymphatic swelling . . . . Lithospermum and Oyster Shell Combination
Menopausal distress . . . . Bupleurum and Peony Formula
Nightsweats . . . . Phellodendron Combination
Obesity (with constipation) . . Siler and Platycodon Combination
Postpartum conditions . . . . . Cnidium and Rehmannia Combination
Premenstrual syndrome . . . . . Bupleurum and Peony Formula
Skin disorders . . . . Pueraria and Carthamus; Tang-kuei and Arctium; Bupleurum and Schizonepeta Combination
Tumors . . . . Angelica and Mastic; Lithosperumum and Oyster Shell

FORMULA INDEX

The following 156 formulas are mentioned in this book. 90 of them can be formed from about 60 based formulas by adding single herb granules. Additional information about these formulas is found in:

Commonly Used Chinese Herb Formulas with Illustrations by Hong-Yen Hsu

Natural Healing with Chinese Herbs by Keisetsu Otsuka, et al.

Chinese Herbology: A Professional Training Program by S. Dharmananda

Achyranthes and Plantago Formula . . . 146
Achyranthes Formula . . . 168
Alisma and Hoelen Combination . . . 176
Anemarrhena, Phellodendron, and Rehmannia Formula . . . 146
Angelica and Mastic Combination . . . **170**
Apricot Seed and Linum Formula . . . 106
Astragalus and Aconite Formula . . . 100
Astragalus and Atractylodes Combination . . . **120**
Atractylodes and Pueraria Formula . . . 71
Aurantium and Pinellia Combination . . . 182
Bamboo and Ginseng Combination . . . **56**
Bamboo and Hoelen Combination . . . 184
Bamboo Leaves and Gypsum Combination . . . 108, 158
Benincasa Combination . . . 161
Bupleurum and Chih-shih Combination . . . 40, **54**
Bupleurum and Cinnamon Combination . . . 37, **38**
Bupleurum and Citrus, Pinellia Combination . . . 60
Bupleurum and Cyperus Combination . . . **40**, 54
Bupleurum and Dragon Bone Combination . . . **46**
Bupleurum and Evodia Combination . . . **64**
Bupleurum and Ginseng Combination . . . **62**
Bupleurum and Hoelen Combination . . . 37, 44, 178
Bupleurum and Magnolia Combination . . . **61**
Bupleurum and Peony Formula . . . **58**, 146

Bupleurum and Pinellia Combination **44**
Bupleurum and Pueraria Combination **50**
Bupleurum and Rehmannia Combination **52**
Bupleurum and Schizonepeta Combination **139**
Bupleurum and Scute Combination 36, 76
Bupleurum and Tang-kuei Combination 58, 60, 62
Bupleurum and Tortoise Shell Combination 54
Bupleurum and Trichosanthes Root Combination 42
Bupleurum Formula **60**
Bupleurum, Chih-shih, and Platycodon Combination 36
Bupleurum, Cinnamon, and Ginger Combination **42**
Bupleurum, Pinellia, and Six Major Herbs Combination 72
Bupleurum, Platycodon, and Gypsum Combination 36
Capillaris and Hoelen Formula 178
Cardamom and Six Major Herbs Combination 72
Chih-chiu and Bupleurum Combination 37
Cinnamon and Anemarrhena Combination **100**, 177
Cinnamon and Atractylodes Combination 177
Cinnamon and Hoelen Formula 162, **164**
Cinnamon and Ma-huang Combination 91
Cinnamon and Persica Combination 164, **168**
Cinnamon Combination 91, 92, 178
Citrus and Crataegus Combination 184
Citrus and Pinellia Combination 56, **184**
Clematis and Stephania Combination **166**
Cnidium and Moutan Combination **156**
Cnidium and Rehmannia Combination **172**
Coix Combination 92, **98**
Coptis and Rhubarb Combination 116
Coptis and Scute Combination **116**, 134, 162
Coptis Combination 76
Cyperus and Cluster Combination 70
Four Major Herbs Combination **70**, 74, 82, 162
Gambir Formula **114**
Gardenia and Hoelen Formula 58
Gardenia and Vitex Combination **134**
Gentiana Combination **122**
Ginger, Cinnamon, and Hoelen Combination 164
Ginseng and Astragalus Combination 70, 72
Ginseng and Atractylodes Formula 70
Ginseng and Bamboo Leaves Combination 37
Ginseng and Gypsum Combination 108

Ginseng and Longan Combination **82**
Ginseng and Tang-kuei Ten Combination **74**, 78, 80
Ginseng and Zizyphus Formula **84**
Ginseng Nutritive Combination 74, **80**
Ginseng Stomach Combination 72
Ginseng, Bupleurum, and Longan Combination 82
Gypsum Combination **108**
Gypsum, Coptis, and Scute Combination 117
Hoelen and Areca Combination 61
Hoelen and Jujube Combination 176
Hoelen and Pinellia Combination 182, 184
Hoelen and Saussurea Combination 178
Hoelen and Schizandra Combination 94
Hoelen Five Herb Formula 44, **178**
Lily Combination **150**
Lithospermum and Oyster Shell Combination **136**
Lonicera and Forsythia Formula **110**
Lotus and Citrus Combination 70, 72
Lycium Formula **148**
Lycium, Chrysanthemum, and Rehmannia Formula 146
Ma-huang and Apricot Seed Combination 91
Ma-huang and Atractylodes Combination 91
Ma-huang and Chiang-huo Combination 100
Ma-huang and Cimicifuga Combination 92
Ma-huang and Coix Combination 91
Ma-huang and Ginkgo Combination **96**
Ma-huang and Magnolia Combination 61
Ma-huang and Morus Formula 96
Ma-huang and Peony Combination 100
Ma-huang Combination 91, 92
Ma-huang, Aconite, and Licorice Combination 91
Ma-huang, Licorice, and Apricot Seed Combination . 61, **91**, 96
Magnolia and Ginger Formula 184
Magnolia and Gypsum Combination **138**
Magnolia and Hoelen Combination 178
Magnolia Five Combination 182
Magnolia Seven Combination 106
Major Blue Dragon Combination 91
Major Bupleurum Combination **48**, 54
Major Rhubarb Combination 106
Major Siler Combination **78**
Minor Blue Dragon Combination 92, **94**

Minor Bupleurum Combination **36**, 44, 76, 92, 178
Minor Rhubarb Combination **106**
Moutan and Persica Combination **161**
Ophiopogon and Asarum Combination **126**
Ophiopogon Combination **158**
Phellodendron Combination **144**
Pinellia and Gastrodia Combination **183**
Pinellia and Ginger Combination 76
Pinellia and Ginseng Six Combination 70, 72
Pinellia and Jujube Combination 185
Pinellia and Magnolia Combination **182**, 185
Pinellia Combination **76**
Pinellia, Atractylodes, and Agastache Formula 73, 185
Platycodon and Fritillaria Combination **152**
Polyporus Combination **181**
Pueraria and Carthamus Combination **124**
Pueraria and Magnolia Combination 92
Pueraria Combination **92**, 112
Pueraria Nasal Combination 92, **112**
Rehmannia and Schizandra Formula 146
Rehmannia Eight Formula 146
Rehmannia Six Formula **146**
Rhubarb and Magnolia Combination 106
Rhubarb and Moutan Combination 161
Saussurea and Cardamon Combination 72
Schizonepeta and Siler Combination 139
Scute and Cimicifuga Combination **132**
Siler and Platycodon Combination **130**
Six Major Herbs Combination 70, **72**, 184
Stephania and Astragalus Combination **180**
Stephania and Hoelen Combination 180
Tang-kuei and Anemarrhena Combination **118**
Tang-kuei and Arctium Formula **128**
Tang-kuei and Atractylodes Combination 162
Tang-kuei and Gardenia Combination 52, 116, 162
Tang-kuei and Gelatin Combination 162
Tang-kuei and Ginseng Eight Combination 70, 74, 162
Tang-kuei and Peony Formula 162
Tang-kuei and Rehmannia Combination **154**
Tang-kuei Eight Herb Combination 136
Tang-kuei Formula 162
Tang-kuei Four Combination . . 70, 74, 116, 134, 139, **162**, 166

Tang-kuei Sixteen Herb Formula **86**
Tu-huo and Pueraria Combination 92
Vitality Combination **176**
Vitality Combination Modified (with ginseng,
schizandra, and ophiopogon) 176

TYPICAL DOSES OF CRUDE HERBS AND CONCENTRATES

The majority of Chinese crude herbs are prescribed in the quantities of:

2-4 grams/daily dose *(Japanese system—used for a long period of time)*

6-12 grams/daily dose *(Chinese system—repeated only a few times)*

Of the herbs mentioned in this book, the following are sometimes used in amounts that provide exceptions to the above rule:

HERBS THAT TEND TO BE USED IN LARGER DOSES
(grams per day, Japanese dosage given)

Alisma:	3-6	Hoelen:	3-6
Bupleurum:	2-7	Ma-huang:	2-6
Coix:	3-8	Rehmannia:	2-6
Gypsum:	3-12	Tang-kuei:	2-5
Ophiopogon:	2-10	Pinellia:	2-6

HERBS THAT TEND TO BE USED IN SMALLER DOSES:

Aconite:	0.5-1	Ginger (dry):	1-3
Carthamus:	1-3	Licorice:	1-3
Coptis:	1-3	Phellodendron	1-3

The amount of any herb to be used in a formula will depend on the relative contribution of the herb to the effect of the complete formula. For a minor contribution, the lower part of the range is used; for a major role, the upper part of the range is used. Also, in very large formulas (that is, large number of herbs), the dose of each individual herb is generally small, while in smaller formulas the dose of each individual herb is generally large. Thus, for most formulas with six or fewer herbs, the dosage is close to the upper end of the range, and for most formulas with 12 or more herbs, the dosage is close to the lower end of the range. The total dosage of herbs used in a formula will depend upon the formula, the severity of the ailment, and the constitution of the individual. In general, the adult dosage of crude herbs is about 20-30 grams/day (Japanese system) or 60-90 grams/day (Chinese system).

In *Commonly Used Herb Formulas With Illustrations* by Dr. Hsu, an estimation of relative proportions of each herb (crude herb) based on the ancient measuring systems is given for each formula; these figures are used here as well. Because of variations in measuring systems during Chinese history, and because some herbs were measured by the piece rather than by weight, these numbers are only approximate. Aside from adjusting the ingredients to be included in a formula, one can adjust the relative proportions of herbs in a formula to make it suitable for the individual who takes the herbs.

The concentrated extract granules produced by Sun Ten are standardized so that the average adult daily dosage for any formula is about 4.5-6.0 grams of granules. On the average, a level teaspoon is about 3.0 grams. The concentration ratio of crude herb weight to granule weight also varies, but is on the average about five or six to one; that is, a 3.0 gram quantity of granules is manufactured from about 15-18 grams of crude herbs. The person who consumes 6.0 grams per day of the concentrate is getting the equivalent of a tea made from 30-36 grams of crude herbs.

To add an herb at the proportion of 3.0 grams/day (a typical amount of crude herb used in a formula) to a granule formula, one would add approximately 10 grams of single herb granules to a packet of 100 grams of base formula. This amount of granule was derived from about 50-60 grams of crude herb and will be consumed during a period of about 18 days (110 grams divided into 18 daily doses of 6 grams each). Thus, the amount of the added crude herb will be about 3.0 grams/day.